Managing Pediatric Foot and Ankle Deformity

Editor

ALICE CHU

FOOT AND ANKLE CLINICS

www.foot.theclinics.com

Consulting Editor
MARK S. MYERSON

December 2015 • Volume 20 • Number 4

ELSEVIER

1600 John F. Kennedy Boulevard • Suite 1800 • Philadelphia, Pennsylvania, 19103-2899

http://www.theclinics.com

FOOT AND ANKLE CLINICS Volume 20, Number 4
December 2015 ISSN 1083-7515, ISBN-13: 978-0-323-40246-0

Editor: Jennifer Flynn-Briggs
Developmental Editor: Meredith Clinton

Foot and Ankle Clinics (ISSN 1083-7515) is published quarterly by Elsevier, Inc., 360 Park Avenue South, New York, NY 10010-1710. Months of issue are March, June, September, and December. Periodicals postage paid at New York, NY, and additional mailing offices. Subscription price per year is $315.00 (US individuals), $421.00 (US institutions), $155.00 (US students), $360.00 (Canadian individuals), $506.00 (Canadian institutions), $215.00 (Canadian students), $460.00 (international individuals), $506.00 (international institutions), and $215.00 (international students). To receive student/resident rate, orders must be accompanied by name of affiliated institution, date of term, and the *signature* of program/residency coordinator on institution letterhead. Orders will be billed at individual rate until proof of status is received. Foreign air speed delivery is included in all *Clinics* subscription prices. All prices are subject to change without notice. **POSTMASTER:** Send address changes to *Foot and Ankle Clinics*, Elsevier Health Sciences Division, Subscription Customer Service, 3251 Riverport Lane, Maryland Heights, MO 63043. **Customer Service: 1-800-654-2452 (US and Canada). From outside of the United States and Canada, call 314-447-8871. Fax: 314-447-8029. E-mail: JournalsCustomerService-usa@ elsevier.com (for print support); JournalsOnlineSupport-usa@elsevier.com (for online support).**

Reprints. For copies of 100 or more, of articles in this publication, please contact the Commercial Reprints Department, Elsevier Inc., 360 Park Avenue South, New York, NY 10010-1710. Tel.: 212-633-3874; Fax: 212-633-3820; E-mail: reprints@elsevier.com.

Contributors

CONSULTING EDITOR

MARK S. MYERSON, MD
Director, Department of Orthopaedic Surgery, Institute for Foot and Ankle Reconstruction, Mercy Hospital, Mercy Medical Center, Baltimore, Maryland

EDITOR

ALICE CHU, MD
Assistant Professor of Orthopaedic Surgery, Divisions of Hand Surgery and Pediatric Orthopaedics, Department of Orthopaedic Surgery, Director, New York Ponseti Clubfoot Center, New York University Hospital for Joint Diseases, New York, New York

AUTHORS

AMIETHAB AIYER, MD
Department of Orthopaedic Surgery, Institute for Foot and Ankle Reconstruction, Mercy Hospital, Mercy Medical Center, Baltimore, Maryland

DAWID BURGER, MD
Department of Orthopaedic Surgery, Institute for Foot and Ankle Reconstruction, Mercy Hospital, Mercy Medical Center, Baltimore, Maryland

ALICE CHU, MD
Assistant Professor of Orthopaedic Surgery, Divisions of Hand Surgery and Pediatric Orthopaedics, Department of Orthopaedic Surgery, Director, New York Ponseti Clubfoot Center, New York University Hospital for Joint Diseases, New York, New York

THOMAS M. COOK, PT, PhD
Professor, Department of Orthopedics and Rehabilitation, Carver College of Medicine and College of Public Health, The University of Iowa, Iowa City, Iowa

FERNANDO FARCETTA, MD
Department of Orthopaedic, AACD – Association for Care of Disabled Child, São Paulo, Brazil

DAVID S. FELDMAN, MD
Professor of Orthopaedic Surgery and Pediatrics, New York University Langone Medical Center, New York, New York

MARA S. KARAMITOPOULOS, MD
Department of Orthopaedic Surgery, Maimonides Medical Center, Maimonides Bone and Joint Center, Brooklyn, New York

JOSEPH J. KRZAK, PhD, PT, PCS
Assistant Professor, Physical Therapy Program, College of Health Sciences, Midwestern University, Downers Grove, Illinois; Physical Therapist, Shriners Hospital for Children, Chicago, Illinois

KEN N. KUO, MD
Chair Professor and Director, Center for Evidence-Based Medicine, Taipei Medical University, Taipei, Taiwan; Department of Orthopaedic Surgery, National Taiwan University Hospital, Taipei, Taiwan; Professor, Department of Orthopaedic Surgery, Rush University Medical Center, Chicago, Illinois

A. NOELLE LARSON, MD
Associate Professor, Department of Orthopedic Surgery, Mayo Clinic, Rochester, Minnesota

WALLACE B. LEHMAN, MD
Professor of Orthopaedic Surgery, Division of Pediatric Orthopaedics, New York University Hospital for Joint Diseases, New York, New York

GABRIEL T. MINDLER, MD
Departments of Pediatric Orthopaedics and Adult Foot and Ankle Surgery, Orthopaedic Hospital Speising, Vienna, Austria

JOSE A. MORCUENDE, MD, PhD
Professor, Department of Orthopedics and Rehabilitation, Carver College of Medicine, The University of Iowa, Iowa City, Iowa

SCOTT J. MUBARAK, MD
Professor of Orthopedics, University of California San Diego; Department of Orthopedics, Rady Children's Hospital, San Diego, California

JOSHUA S. MURPHY, MD
Department of Orthopedics, Rady Children's Hospital, San Diego, California

MARK S. MYERSON, MD
Director, Department of Orthopaedic Surgery, Institute for Foot and Ankle Reconstruction, Mercy Hospital, Mercy Medical Center, Baltimore, Maryland

LANA NIRENSTEIN, MD
Department of Orthopaedic Surgery, Maimonides Medical Center, Brooklyn, New York

MONICA PASCHOAL NOGUEIRA, PhD, MD
Pediatric Orthopaedics, Department of Orthopaedic, HSPE State Public Hospital, São Paulo, Brazil

NORMAN Y. OTSUKA, MD
Chief, Pediatric Orthopaedics, The Children's Hospital at Montefiore; Professor of Orthopaedic Surgery and Pediatrics, Albert Einstein College of Medicine, Bronx, New York

CHRISTOF RADLER, MD
Head of Pediatric Orthopaedic Team; Associate Professor, Departments of Pediatric Orthopaedics and Adult Foot and Ankle Surgery, Orthopaedic Hospital Speising, Vienna, Austria

ABDEL MAJID SHEIKH TAHA, MD
Fellow, Department of Orthopaedic Surgery, New York University Langone Medical Center, New York, New York

PETER A. SMITH, MD
Professor, Department of Orthopaedic Surgery, Rush University Medical Center; Attending Orthopaedic Surgeon, Shriners Hospital for Children, Chicago, Illinois

ALVIN W. SU, MD, PhD
Research Fellow, Department of Orthopedic Surgery, Mayo Clinic, Rochester, Minnesota; School of Medicine, National Yang-Ming University, Beitou, Taipei, Taiwan

STEPHANIE J. SWENSEN, MD
Department of Orthopaedic Surgery, New York University Hospital for Joint Diseases, New York, New York

HAROLD JACOB PIETER VAN BOSSE, MD
Department of Orthopaedic Surgery, Shriners Hospital for Children; Temple University, Philadelphia, Pennsylvania

KUAN-WEN WU, MD
Department of Orthopaedic Surgery, National Taiwan University Hospital, Taipei, Taiwan

ALEXANDRE ZUCCON, MD
Department of Orthopaedic, AACD – Association for Care of Disabled Child, São Paulo, Brazil

Contents

Foot and ankle deformities in cerebral palsy can be effectively treated with surgery. Surgery should be considered in patients with significant deformity and those who have pain or difficulty with orthotic and shoe wear. Equinus contracture of both gastrocnemius and soleus can be treated with open tendoachilles lengthening; ankle valgus with medial epiphysiodesis. Equinovarus is more commonly seen in hemiplegic patients and this deformity can usually be treated with tendon transfers. Triple arthrodesis is an option in children with severe degenerative changes. It is important to address all aspects of the child's pathology at the time of surgical correction.

Calcaneonavicular coalitions are an important cause of adolescent foot pain and deformity. The congenital condition is characterized by an aberrant osseous, cartilaginous, or fibrinous union of the calcaneal and navicular bones. Calcaneonavicular coalitions are the most common form of tarsal coalitions identified within epidemiologic studies. A thorough understanding of this clinically significant entity is important for restoring joint motion and preventing long-term disability.

Talocalcaneal coalitions present with complaints of flatfeet, foot or ankle pain after minor injury, or recurrent ankle sprains. Physical examination findings include limited subtalar motion and prominence inferior to the medial malleolus. Use of computed topography (CT) scans is recommended for preoperative planning. Confirmation of resection with intraoperative CT. Resection of talocalcaneal coalitions with fat-graft interposition has superior results to primary arthrodesis. Improved outcomes have been reported after resection with foot scores averaging 90/100 (AOFAS).

Flatfoot is commonly encountered by pediatric orthopedic surgeons and pediatricians. A paucity of literature exists on how to define a flatfoot. The absence of the medial arch with a valgus hindfoot is the hallmark of this pathology. Flatfoot can be flexible or rigid. This review focuses on the diagnosis and treatment of the flexible flatfoot. Most flatfeet are flexible and clinically asymptomatic, and warrant little intervention. If feet are symptomatic, treatment is needed. Most patients who require treatment improve with foot orthotics and exercises. Only feet resistant to conservative modalities are deemed surgical candidates. The presence of a tight heel cord is often found in patients who fail conservative management.

Current clinical concepts are reviewed regarding the epidemiology, anatomy, evaluation, and treatment of pediatric ankle fractures. Correct diagnosis and management relies on appropriate examination, imaging, and knowledge of fracture patterns specific to children. Treatment is guided by patient history, physical examination, plain film radiographs and, in some instances, computed tomography. Treatment goals are to restore acceptable limb alignment, physeal anatomy, and joint congruency. For high-risk physeal fractures, patients should be monitored for growth disturbance as needed until skeletal maturity.

FOOT AND ANKLE CLINICS

RELATED INTEREST

Emergency Medicine Clinics of North America, May 2015 (Vol. 33, No. 2)
Orthopedic Emergencies
David Della-Giustina and Katja Goldflam, *Editors*
Available at: http://www.emed.theclinics.com

THE CLINICS ARE NOW AVAILABLE ONLINE!
Access your subscription at:
www.theclinics.com

Preface

Managing Pediatric Foot and Ankle Deformity

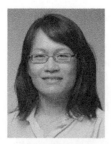

Alice Chu, MD
Editor

This special issue of *Foot and Ankle Clinics of North America* brings together a talented and diverse group of pediatric foot surgeons. I hope that you will find their insights to be helpful to your practice. The topics have been chosen to be those that are either rarely discussed in textbooks, or are relevant enough to require an up-to-date review.

The first group of four articles brings new perspective on clubfoot treatment. First, Jose Morcuende and Thomas Cook describe the obstacles and lessons learned in using the Ponseti method for developing nations. The Ponseti International Association is a great organization that does many wonderful things around the globe. Next, Wallace Lehman and I discuss the challenges facing the practitioner who has already mastered use of the Ponseti method for idiopathic clubfeet. Following this, Cristof Radler and Gabriel Mindler summarize the treatment options for severe recurrent clubfeet, an extremely comprehensive overview. Finally, Dawid Burger, Amiethab Aiyer, and Mark Myerson outline the management of overcorrected clubfoot deformity in adult patients. These are topics that address very complex levels of clubfoot management: how to handle unique complications following Ponseti treatment, how to address complications in childhood as well as overcorrection in adulthood, and how to take the methods we have learned to a global scale.

The next group of four topics has the common theme of foot deformity secondary to pathologic causes. Ken Kuo, Kuan-Wen Wu, Joseph Krzak, and Peter Smith write an overview of common tendon transfers to rebalance dynamic foot deformities. Harold van Bosse narrows the topic to arthrogryposis and myelomeningocele, while Monica Nogueira, Fernando Farcetta, and Alexandre Zuccon illustrate various procedures to correct cavus foot. Last, Mara Karamitopolous and Lana Nirenstein describe core concepts that are critical to solve typical foot problems in patients with spastic cerebral palsy. Although this represents a brief overview of pathologic foot deformities, these four articles represent commonly seen clinical scenarios in pediatric orthopedics.

Foot Ankle Clin N Am 20 (2015) xiii–xiv
http://dx.doi.org/10.1016/j.fcl.2015.09.014
1083-7515/15/$ – see front matter © 2015 Published by Elsevier Inc.

The final four articles are about conditions that are often idiopathic in nature. Stephanie Swensen and Norman Otsuka review the cause and treatment of calcaneonavicular coalitions, while Joshua Murphy and Scott Mubarak present talocalcaneal coalitions. Abdel Majid Sheikh Taha and David Feldman discuss management options for the painful flexible flatfoot. The last article, by Alvin Su and Noelle Larson, is about pediatric ankle fractures, which can help serve as a reminder of the many unique fracture configurations that exist in children.

This issue is informative, thought-provoking, and a great overview of fascinating pediatric foot and ankle problems. I hope you enjoy reading it as much as I did. Many, many thanks to the authors who devoted their time and energy to this endeavor—it is wonderful to have them as friends and colleagues. Finally, a big thank-you to Dr Wallace Lehman, Emeritus Professor of Pediatric Orthoapedic Surgery at NYU–Hospital Joint Diseases, and my fellow director of the New York Ponseti Clubfoot Center. Wally has been my entrée to the world of pediatric foot surgery, and I am forever indebted to him for his guidance and inspiration.

Alice Chu, MD
Department of Orthopaedic Surgery
Division of Pediatric Orthopaedics
Division of Hand Surgery
New York Ponseti Clubfoot Center
NYU–Hospital for Joint Diseases
301 East 17th Street, 4th Floor
New York, NY 10003, USA

E-mail address:
alice.chu@nyumc.org

The Ponseti Method in Low and Middle Income Countries: Challenges and Lessons Learned

Jose A. Morcuende, MD, PhD[a],*, Thomas M. Cook, PT, PhD[b]

KEYWORDS

• Clubfoot • Ponseti method • National programs • Low and middle income countries

KEY POINTS

• Proper training of health professionals and institutionalization of the Ponseti method as the standard of care in the country are critical.
• Successful national programs to treat clubfoot should be based on the core values of high-quality treatment, equitable availability, local direction, and sustainability.
• Experience indicates that the best chances of success in establishing a program include identifying and advising in-country "champions" to provide the leadership, energy, and direction.

INTRODUCTION

Clubfoot is the most common musculoskeletal birth defect in the world. It affects, on average, 1 in every 750 live births, or about 200,000 babies each year worldwide, 80% in low and middle income countries. Additionally, an estimated 1 million individuals are currently living with untreated clubfoot, a rigid, unsightly, lifelong disability that often leads to isolation, abuse, limited access to education, and poverty. Traditional treatment, where available, has been based on major surgical interventions that are very expensive, require highly trained professionals and facilities, and have poor long-term outcomes. In light of these barriers and owing to a lack of awareness and availability regarding a simpler and more cost-effective approach, a high percentage of children are simply left untreated and disabled for life, especially in low and middle income countries.

The Ponseti method is a simple, inexpensive, outpatient treatment that has been proven to be more than 95% effective when properly administered. The Ponseti

The authors' study was supported, in part, by a grant from United States Agency for International Development.
[a] Department of Orthopedics and Rehabilitation, Carver College of Medicine, The University of Iowa, 116 CMAB, Iowa City, IA 52242, USA; [b] Department of Orthopedics and Rehabilitation, Carver College of Medicine and College of Public Health, The University of Iowa, 114 CMAB, Iowa City, IA 52242, USA
* Corresponding author.
E-mail address: Jose-morcuende@uiowa.edu

Foot Ankle Clin N Am 20 (2015) 547–554
http://dx.doi.org/10.1016/j.fcl.2015.07.003
1083-7515/15/$ – see front matter © 2015 Elsevier Inc. All rights reserved.

method is being increasingly adopted in low- and middle-income countries around the world and is the recommended standard for the management of clubfoot. According to a recent article in the *World Journal of Orthopedics*, 113 of the 193 United Nations member countries are currently using the Ponseti method.[1] Although more children born with clubfoot in low- and middle-income countries have access to Ponseti treatment than ever before, the majority of children born with clubfoot in these countries still do not receive access to timely and effective treatment. On average, fewer than 50% of children in low- and middle-income countries are receiving treatment.[2]

The Ponseti International Association (PIA) was established in 2006 to achieve the vision of a world free of untreated clubfoot by training health professionals to apply the Ponseti method and by promoting the institutionalization of this treatment as the standard of care in every country. Four core values guide PIA's efforts. Treatment should be: high quality (rigorously adhering to the Ponseti method), equitable (available to every individual regardless of social or economic status), locally directed (in-country health professionals in charge), and sustainable (integrated into the available health care services using resources from the community and the government).

PIA's experience in more than 50 countries[3–17] has made it clear that establishing sustainable national clubfoot programs requires rigorous training and adoption of the Ponseti method by treatment providers as well as training and facilitation regarding how to strengthen and scale up clubfoot services within the existing health care system.[18,19] A key feature in this approach is the role of in-country "champions" providing the leadership, energy, and direction to build their national program.[20–22] A program champion is someone with a unique combination of skills—passion, persistence, and persuasiveness—who is a respected leader within the health care community and is in a position to influence others. Champions perform a variety of important functions at various levels in building a program, including serving as Ponseti treatment providers, training other providers on the Ponseti method, ensuring quality of treatment, engaging local and national groups to increase awareness and support for the Ponseti method and its institutionalization, and developing the strategic thinking and plans to accomplish all of these tasks.

Another important feature of this approach is the recognition and involvement of stakeholders, defined as any entity with a declared or conceivable interest or stake in a change in policy or practice. This term applies to all individuals and organizations whose commitment and cooperation is required to diffuse the Ponseti-based clubfoot care pathway. Stakeholders are found at all levels of the society, but primarily include health service providers, parents of the children who are beneficiaries of the Ponseti method, health system managers, leaders of professional societies and training institutions, and administrators and policymakers.

The following are some of the key challenges and lessons learned while guiding and supporting in-country champions and other stakeholders to establish and scale up national clubfoot programs in more than 50 low and middle income countries, where health system resources are often limited.

CHALLENGES

As is the case with every instance of diffusion of an innovation,[20] and especially with diffusing a health care innovation[21] in a low-resource environment, there are a number of challenges to be overcome when implementing a national clubfoot program.

Competing Clinical Obligations

Orthopedic surgeons in most low and middle income countries find it difficult to take time away from their clinical duties and to get permission from their supervisors to take time to be mentored in applying the Ponseti method. In many instances, recognition of the value of establishing clubfoot clinical units by the Ministry of Health and/or by the Orthopedic Association is especially helpful in addressing this challenge. Likewise, configuring a mentoring/training program to be condensed into the shortest possible period, rather than requiring multiple short trips over many weeks, can help to overcome this constraint.

Developing a Population Perspective on Managing Clubfoot

Another challenge often encountered by program champions is thinking about clubfoot deformity as a national problem in need of a national solution. Whereas communicable disease doctors and public health professionals are accustomed to dealing with health problems that affect broad populations, most orthopedic surgeons tend to be rather independent in their practices and spend most of their time dealing with individual patients rather than groups of patients. Many have little experience developing strategies for national (public health) approaches. Therefore, it is advantageous to have a group of program champions that includes individuals with experience dealing with health issues on a national scale and experience with promoting national programs.

Engaging Community-Based Organizations

Another issue that can be challenging is engaging stakeholders in support of community-based aspects of a program, including community frontline health workers and, sometimes, local health administrators. This difficulty may be a reflection of the "distance" of some of these stakeholder groups from the day-to-day activities of orthopedic surgeons. For example, reaching out to parent groups and community health workers requires time commitments and relationships that most clinical champions may not possess. Therefore, broadening the project team to include stakeholders who regularly engage these other groups may be one solution to this challenge.

Maintaining Comprehensive Patient Medical Records

High clinical demands on providers' time, unavailability of computer resources at clinical sites, shortage of computer-literate support staff, unreliable electricity, and the high cost of and inconsistent access to the Internet can make it difficult to maintain comprehensive patient medical records. To help overcome this challenge, the PIA and the University of Iowa's Center for Bioinformatics and Computational Biology have developed an International Clubfoot Registry (ICR). The purpose of the registry is to allow health care professionals from around the world to enter data into a standardized electronic medical record system to help ensure the highest quality of treatment and the best possible outcomes. Registry data include an array of indicators, such as the patient's age at initial visit, the number of casts applied to obtain correction, the use of tenotomies, the number of follow-up visits during bracing, and other parameters. Photos of the feet during various stages of treatment are also used to document treatment outcomes. The ICR supports online (PC, Mac, and Linux) and offline (PC currently) data entry capabilities and will soon allow data entry using mobile (Android) devices. The ICR is freely available to any qualified Ponseti treatment provider and is being used currently in more than 587 clinics and hospitals in 44 countries, has more than 516 active users, and contains information from more than 14,609 patients who have made more than 77,674 patient visits (https://icr.uiowa.edu).

Quality and Cost of Braces and Adherence to the Bracing Protocol

Adherence in the use of bracing is a challenge worldwide because the Ponseti method leads to a foot that both appears and functions normally. Parents and caregivers sometimes do not understand fully the need for continued use of a brace and the need for return visits to monitor for relapses. In addition, brace makers in many low and middle income countries have varying levels of expertise and work with locally available materials that often vary widely with regard to quality. In addition, the cost of the braces can vary greatly. Standardization of bracing and bracing protocols for all clinical units in a national program can help to overcome this constraint.

Health System Functionality

A number of issues related to health care systems often add complexity to the task of integrating the clubfoot care pathway into national systems. The Ministry of Health in every low and middle income country is faced with competing demands for limited resources and supporting clubfoot treatment may not be a priority when faced with other, more life-threatening childhood illnesses. Also, in many low-resource countries, there may be frequent changes in leadership within the health system, which adds to the challenges of institutionalizing any health care innovation such as the Ponseti method. However, with the strong commitment of in-country champions and the respective orthopedic associations, champions in many countries have been able to overcome many health system limitations and obtain consistent endorsements and support for the Ponseti method and best practice guidelines for the treatment of clubfoot.

LESSONS LEARNED

In reflecting on experiences in the last 8 years in more than 50 countries, a number of important lessons have been learned about how to diffuse a health care innovation, such as the management of clubfoot using the Ponseti method.

In-Country Champions and Change Agents Are Essential

A proven strategy for building treatment capacity in low-resource settings is to empower in-country "champions" to diffuse a health care innovation. In the case of clubfoot, this has typically been a physician, or other health professional, who has attended a presentation or participated in an introductory course on the Ponseti method and has decided that this treatment method should become the standard of care in his or her facility, region, or country. These individuals can be considered early adopters, those who are eager to try a new idea and rely heavily on their own intuition and vision. Although individuals from a variety of backgrounds may function as champions, our experience indicates that established in-country health professionals usually have the greatest influence with professional colleagues, professional societies, training institutions, and health administrators and health ministries. They also provide credible voices for media outlets and public awareness campaigns. Additionally, parents and family members of affected patients are often strong advocates for continued capacity building, especially once they have first-hand experience with successful treatment.

A Diverse Mix of Skill Sets and Interests Among Champions Is Important

Diverse champion groups are likely to be more effective than those that are more homogeneous, particularly if they include individuals with training and experience in public health and outreach activities. As a recent example,[23] the national program in Pakistan included senior as well as more junior orthopedic surgeons, representatives from different geographic areas of the country, professors and clinicians, officers and former officers in the Pakistan Orthopedic Association, individuals who were well-connected with provincial ministries of health, and those who had knowledge of, and experience with, a population perspective on health issues. This diversity and the ability to divide tasks based on each champion's strengths and interests resulted in successful implementation of the program and a strong foundation on which to sustain program activities and future growth.

Local Stakeholders Should Develop Their Own Vision, Action Plan, and Timelines

A clearly stated, common vision of what will be the outcome of diffusing an innovation is critical to building the various elements of a program. One recent example of a vision statement is, "High quality treatment of clubfoot using the Ponseti method will be available to every child born in our country by 2020." Such a vision statement then leads to the development of timelines, the identification of needs for additional training, the selection of future clinical unit locations, and careful consideration of how to develop and/or strengthen the different aspects required to develop from the start a sustainable program. Simple, easily understood tools like a SWOT analysis (strengths–weakness–opportunities–threats) can be used to support the planning process.[24] The plan needs to be reviewed regularly because circumstances, personnel, and external influences can change frequently, especially in low-resource settings.

Although efforts to build or strengthen several areas of a national program can, and sometimes should, be undertaken concurrently, timing of the development and/or strengthening of the program can be important. In the case of clubfoot, it is important to have well-trained treatment providers, clinical staff, and facilities/supplies in place before the demand for services is generated through public awareness campaigns or policy directives. Substandard, ineffective care by poorly trained providers may not only negatively impact those patients being treated, but can also suppress future referrals and discredit use of an innovation among health professionals and administrators.

Focus on Sustainability from the Beginning

Not seeking funding for patient services from outside the existing health system, as difficult as this might be in some circumstances, promotes the concepts of local ownership and self-determinism. In the case of an innovation like the Ponseti method, which relies primarily on the knowledge and skill of treatment providers and requires relatively low-cost supplies, there may be little, if any, need to provide external financial support for patient care. In a recent United States Agency for International Development (USAID)-supported 2 year project in Pakistan, Nigeria, and Peru,[23] establishing high-quality, equitable, locally directed, and sustainable clubfoot services only required investments in comprehensive training of treatment providers and support and advice for in-country champions to promote the Ponseti method among their peers, professional societies, training institutions, and health administrators. Therefore, the priorities for sources of financial support of clubfoot clinical units should be, first and foremost, the national/state/local health system, followed by national or local nongovernmental organizations, and, then, extranational organizations. In circumstances where resources from external donors are absolutely needed to help establish new services, the underlying principle should be that such support is provided for a clearly defined, time-limited period and with a clear exit strategy.

Linking Clinical and Programmatic Training Enhances Program Development

The majority of the champions who are involved in developing national programs are usually first and foremost skilled clinicians whose primary focus is dealing with orthopedic issues. Given their high clinical demands, the time they have available for meetings and for training activities that take them away from their clinical duties is very limited. Because health care professionals seem most interested in improving their clinical knowledge and skills, and are less familiar with programmatic issues, it is often helpful to combine clinical and programmatic topics in the same meeting. For example, the Advanced Ponseti Workshop in Nigeria in 2014 brought together clinical stakeholders for training on the Ponseti method, but it also introduced them to the Nigeria Sustainable Clubfoot Child Care Program and the concept of a broader national strategy. Because of this combined workshop agenda, several new stakeholders were identified who made commitments to engage in community outreach and awareness activities.

Support by the Orthopedic Society and Ministry of Health Can Accelerate Program Development

A tipping point in the development of a national program is often reached when there is a critical mass of treatment providers who are achieving successful clinical results and the treatment method is then formally endorsed by the country's orthopedic association. Such endorsement then leads to further acceptance within the broader orthopedic community and the inclusion of the Ponseti method in the final orthopedic board examination. As a result, training institutions must provide corresponding training for all residents. These developments often provide the basis for signing a memorandum of understanding with the ministry of health and accelerate the adoption of the best practice guidelines by the ministry. Recognition and adoption of best practice guidelines by the ministry of health can be considered to be a significant milestone in achieving sustainability of the clubfoot care pathway. This development leads to standardization of clubfoot treatment nationally and further institutionalizes the Ponseti method within training programs (physicians, nurses, midwives, etc) and, ultimately, to a reduced burden of disease resulting from clubfoot disability. The end result is in-country sustainable support for clubfoot services. These Best Practice Guidelines for the Management of Clubfoot using the Ponseti method will soon be available for adoption by other countries (http://www.ponseti.info).

SUMMARY

Diffusing a health care innovation like the Ponseti method in low and middle income countries requires more than the application of the traditional continuing medical education approach of providing lectures on the topic. Because of challenges such as limited personnel, competing priorities, inadequate medical supplies, and limited resources, establishing a national program to provide high quality Ponseti management to every child affected by clubfoot requires programmatic thinking and strong leadership. Experience in many countries has indicated that the best chances of success in establishing such a program include identifying and advising in-country "champions" to provide the leadership, energy, and direction to build the program. The lessons that have been learned in applying this approach should be helpful to those who are working to establish a program that is high quality, equitable, locally directed, and meets the criteria for sustainability: integrated into the available health care services, functioning effectively for the foreseeable future, and using resources mobilized by the community and the government.

REFERENCES

1. Shabtai L, Specht SC, Herzenberg JE. Worldwide spread of Ponseti method for clubfeet. World J Orthop 2014;5(5):585–90.

2. Global Clubfoot Initiative. Global Clubfoot Report 2013. Available at: http://globalclubfoot.org/. Accessed March 20, 2015.
3. Palma M, Cook T, Segura J, et al. Barriers to the Ponseti method in Peru: a two-year follow-up. Iowa Orthop J 2013;33:172–7.
4. Nogueira MP, Fox M, Miller K, et al. The Ponseti method of treatment for clubfoot in Brazil: barriers to bracing compliance. Iowa Orthopaedic J 2013;33:161–6.
5. Jayawardena A, Wijayasinghe SR, Tennakoon D, et al. Early effects of a 'train the trainer' approach to Ponseti method dissemination: a case study of Sri Lanka. Iowa Orthopaedic J 2013;33:153–60.
6. Jayawardena A, Zionts LE, Morcuende JA. Management of idiopathic clubfoot after formal training in the Ponseti method: a multi-year, international survey. Iowa Orthopaedic J 2013;33:136–41.
7. Owen RM, Penny JN, Mayo A, et al. A collaborative public health approach to clubfoot intervention in 10 low-income and middle-income countries: 2-year outcomes and lessons learnt. J Pediatr Orthop B 2012;21(4):361–5.
8. Akintayo OA, Adegbehingbe O, Cook T, et al. Initial program evaluation of the Ponseti method in Nigeria. Iowa Orthopaedic J 2012;32:141–9.
9. Adegbehingbe OO, Oginni LM, Ogundele OJ, et al. Ponseti clubfoot management: changing surgical trends in Nigeria. Iowa Orthopaedic J 2010;30:7–14.
10. Gadhok K, Belthur MV, Aroojis AJ, et al. Qualitative assessment of the challenges to the treatment of idiopathic clubfoot by the Ponseti method in urban India. Iowa Orthopaedic J 2012;32:135–40.
11. Wu V, Nguyen M, Nhi HM, et al. Evaluation of the progress and challenges facing the Ponseti method program in Vietnam. Iowa Orthopaedic J 2012;32:125–34.
12. Jayawardena A, Boardman A, Cook T, et al. Diffusion of innovation: onhancing the dissemination of the Ponseti method in Latin America through virtual forums. Iowa Orthopaedic J 2011;31:36–42.
13. Boardman A, Jayawardena A, Oprescu F, et al. The Ponseti method in Latin America: initial impact and barriers to its diffusion and implementation. Iowa Orthopaedic J 2011;31:30–5.
14. Lu N, Zhao L, Du Q, et al. From cutting to casting: impact and initial barriers to the Ponseti method of clubfoot treatment in China. Iowa Orthopaedic J 2010;30:1–6.
15. Palma M, Cook T, Segura J, et al. Descriptive epidemiology of clubfoot in Peru: a clinic-based study. Iowa Orthopaedic J 2013;33:167–71.
16. Nguyen MC, Nhi HM, Nam VQ, et al. Descriptive epidemiology of clubfoot in Vietnam: a clinic-based study. Iowa Orthopaedic J 2012;32:120–4.
17. Pirani S, Naddumba E, Mathias R, et al. Towards effective Ponseti clubfoot care: the Uganda sustainable clubfoot care project. Clin Orthop Relat Res 2009;467:1154–63.
18. Crisp BR, Swerissen H, Duckett S. Four approaches to capacity building in health: consequences for measurement and accountability. Health Promot Int 2000;15(2):99–107.
19. Harmer L, Rhatigan J. Clubfoot care in low-income and middle-income countries: from clinical innovation to public health program. World J Surg 2014;38:839–48.
20. Rogers EM. Diffusion of innovations. New York: The Free Press; 1995.
21. Berwick DM. Disseminating innovations in health care. JAMA 2003;289(15):1969–75.
22. Dearing JW. Applying diffusion of innovation theory to intervention development. Res Soc Work Pract 2009;19:503–18.
23. Morcuende JA, Cook TM, et al. Clubfoot Disability: model for sustainable health systems programs in three countries, United States Agency for International

Development (USAID) under Cooperative Agreement AID-OAA-A-11-00015, February, 2015.

24. Helms MH, Nixon J. Exploring SWOT analysis – where are we now? A review of academic research from the last decade. Journal of Strategy and Management 2010;3(3):215–51.

Treatment of Idiopathic Clubfoot in the Ponseti Era and Beyond

Alice Chu, MD[a,b,*], Wallace B. Lehman, MD[b]

KEYWORDS

- Clubfoot • Talipes equinovarus • Ponseti • History

KEY POINTS

- The Ponseti method has replaced posteromedial release for initial correction of idiopathic clubfoot.
- The Ponseti method has been used successfully, with some modifications, for other types of clubfoot: complex idiopathic, arthrogryposis, myelomeningocele, recurrence after surgery, and neglected/older patients.
- There are new issues raised by this change in treatment.

A SHORT HISTORY OF THE PONSETI METHOD

Over the last several decades, the pendulum of idiopathic clubfoot treatment has swung from nonoperative, to operative, to nonoperative once again.[1] In 1970, Dr Hiram Kite, a proponent of casting, urged "knowledge, patience, and enthusiasm" when correcting clubfeet.[2] His series of infant patients spent an average of 38.4 weeks in casts, which along with poor reproducibility, relegated the technique to the sidelines for most practitioners. In the 1980s and 1990s, surgeons became increasingly aggressive with invasive surgical techniques. A 1991 symposium of international clubfoot surgeons yielded 594 pages devoted to results after surgery, and only 6 pages to nonoperative techniques.[3]

Throughout this period, an orthopedist working at the University of Iowa was also publishing his results using an alternative casting technique. Dr Ignacio Ponseti, a refugee of the Spanish Civil War and a professor of orthopaedic surgery at the University of Iowa, had started the technique in 1948. By 1963, he published on a series of 67

ª Division of Hand Surgery, Department of Orthopaedic Surgery, New York University Hospital for Joint Diseases, 301 E. 17th Street, New York, NY 10003, USA; ᵇ Division of Pediatric Orthopaedics, New York University Hospital for Joint Diseases, 301 E. 17th Street, New York, NY 10003, USA
* Corresponding author. Department of Orthopaedic Surgery, NYU Hospital for Joint Diseases, 301 E. 17th Street, New York, NY 10003.
E-mail address: Alice.Chu@nyumc.org

Foot Ankle Clin N Am 20 (2015) 555–562
http://dx.doi.org/10.1016/j.fcl.2015.08.002
1083-7515/15/$ – see front matter © 2015 Elsevier Inc. All rights reserved.

patients with 5- to 13-year follow-ups, and reported 71% good results after a treatment program of 9.5 weeks of casting.[4] Unfortunately, the timing of this publication coincided with Dr Kite's monograph, and casting for clubfoot was falling into disfavor. Aggressive surgery was producing equally good results, and for a long period of time the trend was toward early posteromedial release after placement of a few initial casts.[3]

As surgeons began to see the final outcomes of surgery at adulthood, there was a growing realization that invasive approaches had major drawbacks. Although results were good during childhood, 10- to 20-year follow-up data showed that patients had premature arthritis, stiffness, and pain.[5,6] There was a possibility of rigid recurrence, as well as overcorrection, and the solutions to these problems were difficult (**Fig. 1**). Additionally, surgery had multiple short-term complications, including avascular necrosis of the talus, wound dehiscence, and infection.[7] In 1995, Cooper and Dietz published a 30-year follow-up study that reported 78% good or excellent results after Ponseti treatment and 1 year later Dr Ponseti published his definitive tome on clubfoot casting.[8,9] The timing was now favorable, and these publications generated significant interest among practitioners treating clubfoot.

Owing to this surge in interest, Dr Ponseti, by then retired from the University of Iowa, conducted many workshops on his technique. Several years later, other centers began reporting similar results, and in the decade from the early 2000s to the present time, the rate of posteromedial release has decreased to almost insignificant numbers.[1] A recent publication comparing long-term results of clubfoot release versus the Ponseti method showed that patients with casting fared better in terms of increased motion, greater strength, and less arthritis.[10]

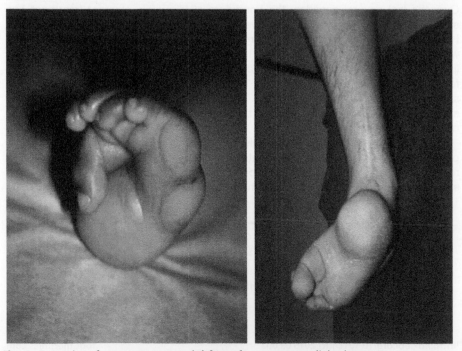

Fig. 1. Examples of severe recurrent clubfeet after posteromedial release.

PEARLS ABOUT PONSETI CASTING

Dr Ponseti contributed several innovative ideas to the method of clubfoot casting. The source of his inspiration may have been personal as well as professional. In his early childhood, he was said to have observed his father, a watchmaker, and he once described the manipulation of clubfoot as being similar to playing "keys on a piano." During his first job as a physician in the Spanish Civil War, Ponseti treated fractures with meticulous casting. He had the experience and conviction to believe that well-molded casts could be used to treat deformity. When he practiced in rural Mexico, Ponseti became acquainted with a man who had a severe disability secondary to failed surgical treatment of clubfoot. Finally, during his residency at the University of Iowa under Dr Arthur Steindler, he was influenced to consider the potential superiority of nonoperative treatment for not only clubfoot, but for disk herniation as well.

In Ponseti's technique, the first cast consists of supination of the forefoot. In this way, the cavus is treated and the forefoot/midfoot unit becomes reduced. The bony congruity between the forefoot and midfoot allows for the unit to be moved en bloc. Subsequent maneuvers consist of abduction or external rotation pressure on the forefoot with counterpressure on the lateral head of the talus. The forefoot/midfoot unit therefore can move the calcaneus from varus to valgus, through indirect pressure, with the talus as the fixed point. The metatarsus adductus and heel varus are corrected simultaneously. Once the heel is in valgus (some care must be taken in very young infants not to overcorrect, although Dr Ponseti did not believe overcorrection was possible) tibiotalar dorsiflexion can be addressed through sequential casts or sectioning of the Achilles tendon (Fig. 2).[8]

When the foot has been corrected, nighttime abduction bracing is instituted for several years. Compliance with bracing is essential for maintenance of correction.[11] The original brace was a static device, but in recent years it has undergone modifications.[12] Initial correction has been reported to be 91% to 100%, but recurrence is

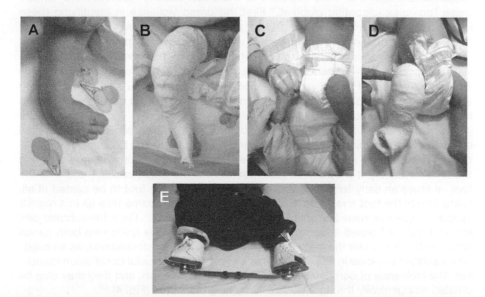

Fig. 2. (A) Idiopathic clubfoot in an infant. (B) First casting maneuver. (C) Percutaneous Achilles tenotomy. (D) Final cast placement. (E) Foot abduction orthosis.

highly possible and strict follow-up is essential to the long-term success of the technique.[13–15] Richards and colleagues[16] reported relapses in 37% of feet treated with the Ponseti method, occurring with a follow-up of 4.3 years. Although many authors have looked at the roles of varying factors, including gender, race, parental marital status, age of patient at the initiation of treatment, number of casts applied, and prior treatment, the only factor consistently noted to be significant is compliance with nighttime bracing.[17] Classification schemes have been used for the initial examination, but have not been found to be useful thereafter (**Fig. 3**).

ETIOLOGY OF IDIOPATHIC CLUBFOOT

Syndromic clubfoot may be seen in patients with distal arthrogryposis, myotonic dystrophy, myelomeningocele, trisomy 18, amniotic band syndrome, or other disorders. In 80% of cases, there is no known associated condition; however, a subclinical disease process has long been suspected.[18] There have been many theories as to the cause of idiopathic clubfoot in patients. Some have considered it to be an arrest in otherwise normal fetal development; others speculated that there were intrinsic abnormalities in the tendon or bone. There are data to support a neuromuscular dysfunction with associated vascular and skeletal changes, although the root cause is uncertain.[19] Because 25% of patients report a positive family history, there is certainly a genetic component. Dobbs and Gurnett[18] have published studies that have led to improved hypotheses. One possible model for clubfoot is a polygenic inheritance model with a dimorphic sex threshold. Genes that have been implicated in the pathway include those in the PITX1–TBX4 transcription pathway.[18]

OTHER DIRECTIONS FOR PONSETI CASTING

A natural progression of a successful technique is to extrapolate it to other purposes through minor modifications. In 2006, Dr Ponseti published on a series of seemingly idiopathic clubfoot that were resistant to the usual casting method.[20] He termed these "complex idiopathic clubfeet." First, he urged vigilance in identifying these feet, which he described as being short and stubby, with severe equinus of the heel, plantarflexion of the metatarsals, a deep transverse plantar crease, and apparent shortening and hyperextension of the big toe. This type of foot typically resists casting, and the continued slippage causes worsening of the deformity. To secure the cast, Dr Ponseti recommended hyperflexion of the knee to 110°, with anterior knee and posterior ankle splints. In the same article, he described a revised manipulation technique.

The manipulation consists of the usual supination maneuver followed by adduction of the forefoot and midfoot around the lateral head of the talus. Because of the difficulty in palpating the subtalar joint, Dr Ponseti emphasized the importance of taking the time to identify it properly. In fact, because of the short, stubby nature of the foot, at times an early tenotomy was necessary to allow the foot to be casted at all. Adduction of the foot should be able to be corrected in the same time as in a regular idiopathic foot, but these feet should not be abducted past 40°. Once the subtalar joint is corrected, Dr Ponseti described "grasping the foot by the ankle with both hands while the thumbs under the metatarsals pushed the foot into dorsiflexion, as an assistant stabilized the knee in flexion"; in other words, a fairly forceful dorsiflexion maneuver. The incidence of complex idiopathic clubfeet is unknown, and they may also be created iatrogenically through a failure of casting technique (**Fig. 4**).[20]

Other modifications have since been made and the indications have been broadened. The Ponseti technique has been used successfully in patients with

Clubfoot Center
Visit Worksheet

Date_____

Name_____ Foot (circle): R   L

<u>**Current Cast Number**</u> (circle): 0 1 2 3 4 5 6 7 8 9 ___   <u>**Atypical**</u> (circle if yes)

<u>**Complications**</u> (circle) 0)None 1)Rocker sole 2)Maceration 3)Abrasion 4)Blister 5)Slough 6)Decubitus
        7)Cast saw injury 8)Cast intolerance/removal 9)Cast fell off 10)Other_____

<u>**Surgical Date:**</u> _____**Procedure:** (circle) 1)None 2)Per-Q Achilles tenotomy 3)Open TAL/post release
                        4)PMR 5)Anterior tibialis transfer 6)Other_____

<u>**Date DBB Applied:**</u> _____**Compliance:** 1) YES 2) NO   **Wearing**: 1) Full time 2) Night/Naptime
                        Age bar stopped at: ___yrs ___mos   **Stopped by:** 1) MD 2)Parents

<u>**Dimeglio/Bensahel**</u>

1. Equinus	Points		Points	For parts 5–8, Mark Points as Present = 1, Absent = 0	Points
Dorsiflexion _____°		**3. Midfoot Rotation (Horizontal plane)**			
Plantarflexion 45°–90°	4	Supination 45°–90°	4	**5. Posterior Crease**	
Plantarflexion 20°–45°	3	Supination 20°–45°	3	**6. Medial Crease**	
Plantarflexion 0°–20°	2	Supination 0°–20°	2	**7. Cavus**	
Dorsiflexion 20°–0°	1	Pronation 20°–0°	1	**8. Abnormal underlying musculature**	
Dorsiflexion >20°	0	Pronation >20°	0		
2. Hindfoot varus		**4. Forefoot Adduction (on hindfoot)**			
Varus 45°–90°	4	Adductus 45°–90°	4	**TOTAL SCORE**	
Varus 20°–45°	3	Adductus 20°–45°	3	Type I: 0– 5 points	
Varus 0°–20°	2	Adductus 0°–20°	2	Type IIa: 6–10 points	
Valgus 20°–0°	1	Abductus 20°– 0°	1	Type IIb: 11–15 points	
Valgus >20°	0	Abductus >20°	0	Type III: 16–20 points	

<u>**Catterall/Pirani (Normal: 0 points; most abnormal 1.0 points)**</u>

Hindfoot contracture (HFCS)	Points	Midfoot contracture (MFCS)	Points
a. Posterior crease: 0, 0.5, or 1.0 points		a. Curvature of lateral border: 0, 0.5 or 1.0	
b. Empty heel: 0, 0.5 or 1.0 points		b. Medial crease: 0, 0.5 or 1.0 points	
c. Rigid equinus: 0, 0.5 or 1.0 points		c. Lateral head of talus: 0, 0.5, or 1.0 points	
HFCS Sub-total		**MFCS Sub-total**		**Total Score (HFCS and MFCS)**	

Dorsiflexion X-rays:

<u>**PLAN:**</u> ☐ Recast   ☐ X-ray on follow-up   ☐ Photograph   ☐ Follow-up ___ wk(s)

Signed:

Fig. 3. Form with Dimeglio/Bensahel and Catterall/Pirani scoring systems. (*From* Chu A, Labar AS, Sala DA, et al. Clubfoot classification: correlation with Ponseti cast treatment. J Pediatr Orthop 2010;30:696; with permission.)

arthrogryposis, myelomeningocele, recurrence after posteromedial release, and neglected clubfeet.[21–25] The outcomes after casting in arthrogryposis and myelomeningocele are discussed in Syndromic Feet: Arthrogryposis and Myelomeningocele by Harold Jacob Pieter van Bosse.[26] In children who have recurrences after prior

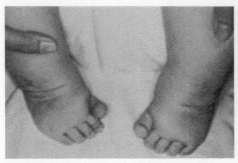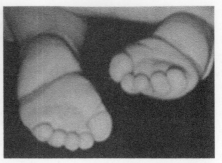

Fig. 4. Complex idiopathic clubfoot. (*From* Chu A and Lehman WB, Persistent clubfoot deformity following treatment by the Ponseti method. J Pediatr Orthop 2012;21:41; with permission.)

surgery, a series of 58 children (83 clubfeet) with an average age of 5 years, 2 months showed successful attainment of plantigrade feet in 86% of cases.[22] The authors did not modify the technique in that study, and they required an average of 4 casts. Neglected clubfeet in older individuals have also been treated with the Ponseti method with satisfactory results.[27]

Morcuende and colleagues[28] have also published on an accelerated casting regimen that can shorten the time needed for initial treatment. Instead of weekly cast changes, the time between casts was decreased to 5 days. The results in that series showed no difference between the 7- and 5-day groups with respect to the number of casts required for full correction.

Congenital vertical talus has been treated with a casting methodology similar to the Ponseti method performed in reverse.[29] The core principles of the Ponseti method seem to be highly effective for treating idiopathic as well as syndromic congenital foot disorders, and continue to be extrapolated to other areas by other practioners.[30]

THE "POST-PONSETI ERA"

Many authors have now reported excellent initial outcomes after use of the Ponseti method in idiopathic clubfoot. However, relapse rates occur in approximately 30% of cases, and these numbers depend significantly on compliance with a very long period of bracing.[31] Now that the Ponseti method for initial clubfoot treatment has been accepted widely, several questions have arisen.[32] How to manage relapses after Ponseti treatment? (How is this similar or different to managing recurrence after surgical treatment?) How to track and successfully institute parental compliance with bracing. What are alternatives to bracing?

Richards noted that one-third of post-Ponseti relapses could be treated nonoperatively, whereas the remaining two-thirds were treated surgically.[16] In the absence of static deformity, a tibialis anterior tendon transfer has excellent long-term results in preventing additional deformity without affecting function.[33] More information on this topic can be found in Tendon Transfers Around the Foot: When and Where by Ken N Kuo, Kuan-Wen Wu, Joseph J Krzak, and Peter A Smith.[34]

Finally, one wonders if the pendulum has swung so dramatically from operative to nonoperative treatment of clubfoot that it has produced a generation of orthopaedic surgeons who have extremely limited experience with posteromedial release surgery. Although surgery is becoming rare, there will undoubtedly be cases in which it would produce the best result for that particular patient. Some examples would be the rare individual who is completely refractory to casting, or a patient with medical or family issues that make multiple cast changes impossible to perform safely. Indications for the Ponseti method have been broadened to such an extent that teenagers with neglected clubfeet are being casted, which can take months of casting.[27] Is the potential morbidity from 4 months of casting and immobilization worth the decreased surgical rate, or in fact worth the morbidity of a neglected clubfoot? Or would a 1-stage surgery with or without the potential complications be worth it, in those cases? And if so, who has the experience to do the surgery now that the rate of surgery has diminished so dramatically?

SUMMARY

In the past few decades, the Ponseti method has effected a dramatic change in the landscape of clubfoot treatment. It has quite clearly led to excellent results in the short term, and with appropriate treatment of recurrences in the first 5 to 6 years, it can produce improved long-term results when compared with surgery. Using the principles of the Ponseti method, there will be continued innovation and future changes in the landscape of clubfoot treatment as it presently stands.

REFERENCES

1. Zionts LE, Zhao G, Hitchcock K, et al. Has the rate of extensive surgery to treat idiopathic clubfoot declined in the United States? J Bone Joint Surg Am 2010; 92(4):882–9.
2. Kite JH. Conservative treatment of the resistant recurrent clubfoot. Clin Orthop Relat Res 1970;70:93–110.
3. Simons GE. The clubfoot. New York: Springer-Verlag; 1994.
4. Ponseti IV, Smoley EN. The classic: congenital club foot: the results of treatment. 1963. Clin Orthop Relat Res 2009;467(5):1133–45.
5. Aronson J, Puskarich CL. Deformity and disability from treated clubfoot. J Pediatr Orthop 1990;10(1):109–19.
6. Graf A, Hassani S, Krzak J, et al. Long-term outcome evaluation in young adults following clubfoot surgical release. J Pediatr Orthop 2010;30(4):379–85.
7. Herzenberg JE, Radler C, Bor N. Ponseti versus traditional methods of casting for idiopathic clubfoot. J Pediatr Orthop 2002;22(4):517–21.
8. Ponseti IV. Congenital clubfoot: fundamentals of treatment. New York: Oxford University Press; 1996.
9. Cooper DM, Dietz FR. Treatment of idiopathic clubfoot. A thirty-year follow-up note. J Bone Joint Surg Am 1995;77(10):1477–89.
10. Smith PA, Kuo KN, Graf AN, et al. Long-term results of comprehensive clubfoot release versus the Ponseti method: which is better? Clin Orthop Relat Res 2014;472(4):1281–90.
11. Dobbs MB, Rudzki JR, Purcell DB, et al. Factors predictive of outcome after use of the Ponseti method for the treatment of idiopathic clubfeet. J Bone Joint Surg Am 2004;86-A(1):22–7.
12. Chen RC, Gordon JE, Luhmann SJ, et al. A new dynamic foot abduction orthosis for clubfoot treatment. J Pediatr Orthop 2007;27(5):522–8.
13. Abdelgawad AA, Lehman WB, van Bosse HJ, et al. Treatment of idiopathic clubfoot using the Ponseti method: minimum 2-year follow-up. J Pediatr Orthop 2007; 16(2):98–105.
14. Bor N, Herzenberg JE, Frick SL. Ponseti management of clubfoot in older infants. Clin Orthop Relat Res 2006;444:224–8.

15. Radler C, Mindler GT, Riedl K, et al. Midterm results of the Ponseti method in the treatment of congenital clubfoot. Int Orthop 2013;37(9):1827–31.
16. Richards BS, Faulks S, Rathjen KE, et al. A comparison of two nonoperative methods of idiopathic clubfoot correction: the Ponseti method and the French functional (physiotherapy) method. J Bone Joint Surg Am 2008;90(11):2313–21.
17. Chu A, Labar AS, Sala DA, et al. Clubfoot classification: correlation with Ponseti cast treatment. J Pediatr Orthop 2010;30(7):695–9.
18. Dobbs MB, Gurnett CA. Genetics of clubfoot. J Pediatr Orthop 2012;21(1):7–9.
19. Handelsman JE, Badalamente MA. Club foot: a neuromuscular disease. Dev Med Child Neurol 1982;24(1):3–12.
20. Ponseti IV, Zhivkov M, Davis N, et al. Treatment of the complex idiopathic clubfoot. Clin Orthop Relat Res 2006;451:171–6.
21. Van Bosse HJ, Marangoz S, Lehman WB, et al. Correction of arthrogrypotic clubfoot with a modified Ponseti technique. Clin Orthop Relat Res 2009;467(5):1283–93.
22. Nogueira MP, Ey Batlle AM, Alves CG. Is it possible to treat recurrent clubfoot with the Ponseti technique after posteromedial release?: a preliminary study. Clin Orthop Relat Res 2009;467(5):1298–305.
23. Gerlach DJ, Gurnett CA, Limpaphayom N, et al. Early results of the Ponseti method for the treatment of clubfoot associated with myelomeningocele. J Bone Joint Surg Am 2009;91(6):1350–9.
24. Boehm S, Limpaphayom N, Alaee F, et al. Early results of the Ponseti method for the treatment of clubfoot in distal arthrogryposis. J Bone Joint Surg Am 2008;90(7):1501–7.
25. Morcuende JA, Dobbs MB, Frick SL. Results of the Ponseti method in patients with clubfoot associated with arthrogryposis. Iowa Orthop J 2008;28:22–6.
26. van Bosse HJP. Syndromic feet: arthrogryposis and myelomeningocele. Foot Ankle N Am 2015;20(4):619–44.
27. Lourenco AF, Morcuende JA. Correction of neglected idiopathic club foot by the Ponseti method. J Bone Joint Surg Br 2007;89(3):378–81.
28. Morcuende JA, Abbasi D, Dolan LA, et al. Results of an accelerated Ponseti protocol for clubfoot. J Pediatr Orthop 2005;25(5):623–6.
29. Dobbs MB, Purcell DB, Nunley R, et al. Early results of a new method of treatment for idiopathic congenital vertical talus. J Bone Joint Surg Am 2006;88(6):1192–200.
30. Tripathy SK, Saini R, Sudes P, et al. Application of the Ponseti principle for deformity correction in neglected and relapsed clubfoot using the Ilizarov fixator. J Pediatr Orthop B 2011;20(1):26–32.
31. Thacker MM, Scher DM, Sala DA, et al. Use of the foot abduction orthosis following Ponseti casts: is it essential? J Pediatr Orthop 2005;25(2):225–8.
32. Chu A, Lehman WB. Persistent clubfoot deformity following treatment by the Ponseti method. J Pediatr Orthop B 2012;21(1):40–6.
33. Holt JB, Oji DE, Yack HJ, et al. Long-term results of tibialis anterior tendon transfer for relapsed idiopathic clubfoot treated with the Ponseti method: a follow-up of thirty-seven to fifty-five years. J Bone Joint Surg Am 2015;97(1):47–55.
34. Kuo KN, Wu K-W, Krzak JJ, et al. Tendon transfers around the foot: when and where. Foot Ankle Clin N Am 2015.

Treatment of Severe Recurrent Clubfoot

Christof Radler, MD*, Gabriel T. Mindler, MD

KEYWORDS

- Clubfoot • Surgery • Pes equinovarus • Pediatric foot deformity
- Clubfoot recurrence • External fixation

KEY POINTS

- Treatment of severe recurrent clubfoot deformity, especially after previous open release surgeries, can still be challenging.
- Most clubfoot recurrences can be treated using the Ponseti method; only the most rigid and deformed feet in children and young adults need more invasive interventions to obtain good foot function.
- Numerous surgical procedures have been described in the literature over the last century, with many rendered obsolete and most resulting in stiff feet with limited function.
- Indicating the right treatment and surgical procedure is crucial and should always be guided by individual patient needs and functional considerations.

A video that shows postoperative results of a patient diagnosed with fixed equinus accompanies this article at http://www.foot.theclinics.com/

INTRODUCTION

Clubfoot surgery has a long and comprehensive history[1] and the treatment of congenital clubfoot has challenged the orthopedic surgeon throughout the centuries. Surgical correction and interventions have been developed and evolved at the beginning of the 20th century related to improvements and safety of general anesthesia. As a result, nonoperative and minimally invasive techniques were abandoned as outdated, time consuming, and insufficient. At the height of this development, extensive soft tissue releases have been performed in infants often age 3 to 6 months with various

Dr C. Radler is a Consultant for both Smith & Nephew Europe, and Ellipse Inc. Dr G.T. Mindler has nothing to disclose.
Department of Pediatric Orthopaedics and Adult Foot and Ankle Surgery, Orthopaedic Hospital Speising, Speisinger Straße 109, Vienna A 1130, Austria
* Corresponding author. Department of Pediatric Orthopaedics, Orthopaedic Hospital Speising, Speisinger Straße 109, Vienna A 1130, Austria.
E-mail address: christof.radler@oss.at

Foot Ankle Clin N Am 20 (2015) 563–586
http://dx.doi.org/10.1016/j.fcl.2015.07.002
1083-7515/15/$ – see front matter © 2015 Elsevier Inc. All rights reserved.

foot.theclinics.com

approaches and techniques.[2–4] Long-term follow-up diminished the results of these extensive operations, in part because scarring and early arthrosis have been recognized as the most common long-term complications.[5–7] However, failure was not only seen in the long term. Major complications were also met during or after surgery. Failed correction, wound breakdown, skin necrosis, and overcorrection, growth disturbance with massive shortening of the foot and leg were encountered.[8]

These complications and the disappointing long-term outcomes resulted in a reevaluation of clubfoot treatment and a turn toward a less invasive method using detailed serial casting that has already proven effective.[9–12] Doubted by many and suspiciously eyed by others, the rediscovery and rise of the Ponseti method for clubfoot treatment has changed the approach to clubfoot fundamentally. In the meantime, there is a worldwide spread of the Ponseti treatment.[13] With proper casting technique, the right timing and indication for percutaneous Achilles tendon lengthening, optimal support to ensure bracing compliance, frequent follow-up to detect early recurrence, and treatment of recurrence with casting and/or tendon transfers, open joint surgery can be avoided in almost all cases of congenital idiopathic clubfoot,[14] and with good functional outcome.[15] Today the Ponseti method has become the gold standard treatment for congenital clubfoot and the number of operative procedures has decreased significantly.[10,16]

The Ponseti method is additionally applied to persistent, residual, and recurrent clubfoot.[17,18] Tibialis anterior tendon transfer (TATT) with or without prior casting, and with or without percutaneous Achilles lengthening, is the treatment of choice for recurrent or late presenting clubfoot.

Because almost all clubfoot deformities and recurrences can be treated successfully with the Ponseti method, extensive operative interventions have become mostly obsolete and are on the verge of extinction. For the sake of functional clubfoot treatment, this is a highly positive development. However, it has the potential to become a problem for the very few recurrent, neglected, previously operated, or syndromic cases that cannot be managed sufficiently with the Ponseti method. Those cases are usually feet after previous extensive surgery, severe stiff recurrences owing to lack of follow-up, nonidiopathic clubfoot, and stiff residual clubfoot components in children and young adult (**Box 1**). This overview on the treatment of severe recurrent clubfoot discusses the different aspects and pathoanatomy of the recurrent clubfoot and describes the treatment options according to the deformity.

DEFINITION OF SEVERE RECURRENCE

Deformity in previously treated clubfoot is usually defined as residual/resistant or recurrent/relapsed. Although residual deformities are those that have never been corrected,

---

Box 1
Biggest challenges in clubfoot surgery

- Defining a realistic goal of treatment.
- Indicating the individual best treatment approach.
- Low frequency of the procedures owing to the extremely rare indication for open surgery.
- Stiffness in feet that are nonresponsive to the Ponseti method is also a challenge for open surgery.
- Diminishing experience with operative techniques for correction of clubfoot.

recurrence defines deformities that have been fully corrected previously. Detailed and reproducible documentation is the only way to point out cases with insufficient initial correction or factors that might have contributed to recurrence. In daily clinical practice, this differentiation can be difficult, especially in patients treated elsewhere, and even in the literature those cases are often intermixed. The implication of this differentiation on further treatment is often minimal. Nevertheless, in late recurrence of clubfoot deformities, neurologic evaluation should be obtained for search of previously undiagnosed neurologic disease. Lovell and Morcuende[19] found neuromuscular disease in 33% of patients over age 7 presenting with a late relapse. In another series, neuromuscular disease was found in 2 of 10 recurrences after TATT.[20] Further soft tissue abnormalities in treatment-resistant clubfeet have been shown using MRI.[21]

Another entity is neglected clubfoot. These feet were by definition never treated. They often show severe deformity with skin callus on the lateral foot or even on the talar head. Nevertheless, these untouched feet do not present with severe scarring and postoperative degenerations, and many can be treated with the Ponseti method, even in older children.[22–24]

It is not well-defined what constitutes severe recurrence. Is a fast progressive recurrence "severe"? Does it describe the position of the foot or the stiffness of the deformity? Is every clubfoot recurrence in need of surgical correction severe? Scores that describe the initial clubfoot deformity like the Pirani[25] or Dimeglio score[26] and scores for evaluation during growth[27] are not or only partially useful for recurrence in children after walking age. For patients younger than age 7 with recurrence after Ponseti treatment, a classification was described recently,[28] but has not been validated or used widely. Only for older patients or feet after surgical treatment with recurrence no such classification exists.[27] One problem might be the very heterogenic picture of recurrence, especially after open surgery. In those cases, the components of clubfoot that recurred often depend on the initial procedure performed. Combinations of recurrences with residual components can be seen, such as equinus in feet where subtalar correction has never been achieved. Surgically treated feet can additionally show components of iatrogenic deformity.

Severity should not be defined by the ability to correct the deformity using the Ponseti method, because this seems very subjective and is related largely to the experience in and dedication to detailed Ponseti casting.

Initial casting is recommended in all cases independent of severity or age. Even very severe and stiff feet can start to respond after 2 to 3 casts and, if a sufficient correction is not possible, the severity of the deformity can usually be decreased, with the aim of minimizing the surgical approach (Box 2).

CLINICAL ASSESSMENT

A comprehensive clinical assessment and evaluation of complaints and impairments in daily life are the cornerstones of establishing valid treatment goals. The patient's

---

Box 2
Challenging clubfoot feet

- Severe stiff recurrence owing to lack of follow-up.
- Clubfoot recurrence after previous extensive surgery.
- Stiff residual clubfoot deformity after incomplete initial correction or surgery.
- Stiff syndromic clubfoot recurrence.

activity level should be explored and a discussion of limitations and pain with the performed or desired activities should follow. Especially in older children, where a full correction of the deformity is no longer achievable, the focus must be set on function and pain, whereas foot-form and radiographs are secondary objectives.

In clinical gait analysis, initial contact (heel, midfoot, or forefoot) should be examined. Heel position in loading, initial contact, and swing phase can point toward fixed or dynamic varus. Forefoot supination and or adduction can be dynamic because of relative tibialis anterior overpowering, or static in fixed deformities. The foot progression angle, mostly the amount of in-toeing, can be assessed clinically. Care must be taken to differentiate the level of internal rotation. It has been shown that in-toeing in clubfoot is usually not related to internal tibial torsion, but rather to incomplete calcaneal subtalar correction and forefoot adduction.[29]

Compensation mechanisms like hyperextension of the knee joint in the presence of equinus or external hip rotation seen with in-toeing should be noted.[15] If instrumented 3-dimensional gait analysis is not available, a video recording and evaluation in slow motion can facilitate the gait analysis. The important supportive role of gait analysis for preoperative planning was shown in a study by Sankar and colleagues.[30] Preoperative gait analysis resulted in changes of the planned surgical intervention in 19 of 30 patients (63%) with recurrent clubfoot.[30]

The sole of the foot can be examined for calloused skin, and dust or dirt (depending on your clinic floor), which can show areas of plantar contact. Pedobarography can add additional objective information on plantar pressure distribution.

Clinical examination in standing includes the heel position and foot loading as well as discrepancies in leg length, foot length, and foot height. Standing on tiptoes and walking on heels can be tested.

Further examination of clubfoot includes evaluation of active dorsiflexion and plantarflexion and the activity of the tibialis anterior and posterior muscles and the peroneal muscles. Maximal passive ankle dorsiflexion and plantarflexion must be recorded in the extended and flexed knee positions. The subtalar joint must be palpated and examined regarding the reposition of the talar head. After stabilizing the talus, the amount of abduction of the calcaneus from underneath the talus can be palpated. Eversion and inversion of the subtalar joint must be noted. The position and flexibility of the midfoot and forefoot and toe contractures or deformities should be documented as well as the sensibility and recapillarization of the toes. Existing scars must be evaluated and image documented, because skin breakdown or secondary wound healing are likely after repeat surgery. In multiple or extensively operated feet, a vascular status with Doppler ultrasonography or MRI angiography should be considered.

Radiographic Assessment

Computed tomography or MRI are important tools for preoperative planning and the evaluation of osteoarthritis and bony anatomy, depending on the complexity of the case and the age of the patient. However, the main criteria for the selection of an operative procedure remain the hands-on clinical examination and patients' expectations and needs.

Radiographs of the foot anteroposterior and lateral in standing position and lateral maximum dorsiflexion views should be performed. In the presence of adduction and or subtalar internal rotation, the ankle joint is usually not targeted truly lateral and evaluation of the talar dome is not valid. Therefore, a mortise view of the ankle should be added if information on the talar dome is desired.

Computed tomography with or without 3-dimensional reconstruction should be reserved for only the most complex deformities in older children owing to the high dose of radiation. MRI can give information on joint status and detect soft tissue pathologies and areas of overuse in case of pain.

In children and adolescents undergoing extensive surgical correction or especially before external fixation for clubfoot treatment, psychological counseling should be performed preoperatively.

TREATMENT ACCORDING TO PATHOANATOMY

The crucial step to understanding the pathoanatomy is the assessment of the subtalar derotation of the calcaneus. Subtalar derotation is the key to true correction of clubfoot deformity and is usually achieved by the initial Ponseti casting. Without subtalar correction, the heel stays in varus, and the calcaneus and with it the whole foot stays in adduction and supination. The first ray is often plantar flexed and shortened as a compensatory mechanism where the forefoot/midfoot pronates to allow contact of the first metatarsal. Sometimes, this can also be the result of residual cavus or iatrogenic after pronation during correction.

SUBTALAR ROTATION

In recurrence and residual cases, the subtalar correction can again be achieved by casting according to the Ponseti method. Heel valgus and abduction of the calcaneus from underneath the talus are obtained, resulting in divergence between the talus and calcaneus both clinically and radiologically. If necessary, additional Achilles lengthening procedures and/or a TATT can complete the correction.

If subtalar derotation cannot be achieved with casting, other methods are a soft tissue release or gradual correction with external fixation. The most important question at that point is whether repeat surgery is, with all its potential risks, pitfalls, scarring and induction of arthritic changes, a worthwhile endeavor? In certain patients, subtalar derotation is not possible and/or no longer intended. In our experience, this is mostly the case in patients over the age of about 6 to 8 years when a functional subtalar joint can no longer be expected and where it is easier to correct around the true pathology. Additionally, there are feet with sufficient subtalar correction but residual deformities of the forefoot and midfoot or presenting with equinus. In these feet, the main pathologies preventing good function and patient satisfaction can be corrected individually without reducing the subtalar joint.

Correction of the subtalar rotation was classically achieved by extensive soft tissue releases in the pre-Ponseti era,[2–4] with disappointing long term results.[5–7] Even in one of the most recent studies of clubfoot treated with complete subtalar release at age 8 months to 10 years, foot pain was found in 55% of the children at the 9-year follow-up.[31]

Soft tissue releases have been recommended for clubfoot recurrences in children up to age 10 years.[32,33] However, the incongruence of the subtalar joint in such long-standing deformities might lead to a high rate of insufficient correction and arthrosis, in addition to all other sequelae of open joint surgery.

Complete soft tissue clubfoot release has, therefore, been recommended for recurrence up to the age of 4 years by Simons[3] and up to the age of 6 years by Turco.[4] In a different article, Turco stated that, "The best results with the least complications were in children who were operated on between the ages of one and two years."[34] However, this is an age group that can be exclusively and very well-managed with the Ponseti method. Furthermore, he did not recommend his release surgery in older children because "adaptive changes in the shape and articular surfaces of the tarsal bones by that age prevent reduction of the talus into the ankle mortise and reduction of the talo-calcaneonavicular dislocation."[4]

In multiply operated clubfoot not responding to Ponseti casting, another soft tissue release has a very high complication rate with the risk of vascular problems, wound breakdown, and wound healing problems and is again hardly ever indicated. Turco reported the most difficult operations and the poorest results in feet where a prior posterior medial release had been attempted.[4]

Skin problems are a typical complication in extensive soft tissue releases. Different methods to avoid or treat skin necrosis in clubfoot surgery have been reported like serial postoperative casts,[35] local flaps,[36] free gracilis muscle flaps,[37] and different types of surgical incisions.[38] We should bear in mind that these treatments put an enormous physical and psychological burden on the child and family and should be avoided at all cost. In summary, open release surgery is hardly ever indicated in idiopathic clubfoot and very rarely in syndromic or secondary clubfoot and has been mostly abandoned for good.

External fixation has traditionally been recommended for severe recurrences and especially for feet where open surgery was not an option.[39–44] Subtalar derotation can be achieved with an Ilizarov ring fixator with 2 wires that pass through the head of the talus with an olive wire on the lateral side to stabilize the talus during correction.[45]

Lamm and coworkers[46] combined the principle of fixing the talus during subtalar abduction with the use of a hexapod external fixator (Taylor spatial frame, Smith and Nephew, Inc, London, UK) for correction of neglected or relapsed clubfoot. The talus wire is attached to the proximal ring on the tibia during external rotation of the subtalar footplate including some correction of inversion (varus) and subtalar dorsiflexion (Fig. 1). Afterward, the wire stabilizing the talus is detached from the tibial ring and attached to the foot ring. This allows dorsiflexion including some distraction of the ankle joint to obtain overcorrection.[47]

In the presence of adduction and supination as part of the clubfoot deformity, preoperative Ponseti casting can improve the forefoot position to facilitate the frame construction. If this is not possible, the foot ring of the frame has to be cut and turned into an unconstrained frame. This whole technique of correction needs good experience with clubfoot deformity, external fixation, and the use of the Taylor spatial frame. Great experience and care must go into the programming of the prescription for strut adjustments because minor errors can lead to impingement between bones and crushing of cartilage. During distraction of the ankle joint necessary for correction, epiphysiolysis of the distal tibial epiphysis can occur and has been reported for Ilizarov frame treatment.[41,48–50]

Again, the indications for this technique are very limited, because younger patients can sufficiently corrected with casting and patients older than 6 to 8 years have a higher rate of recurrence with soft tissue distraction only, owing to lack of remodeling of the joint surfaces. With no case series reported for this subtalar derotation technique with external fixation, the actual rate of recurrence and functional outcomes are unknown.

If subtalar correction is not performed, the severe recurrent clubfoot can be treated by addressing individual components of the deformity in a multiple step surgery, after once again maximal soft tissue stretch has been achieved by casting.

EQUINUS

Even in well-treated clubfoot, reduced ankle dorsiflexion is a common observation. Equinus recurrence can occur in insufficient initial correction (like incomplete

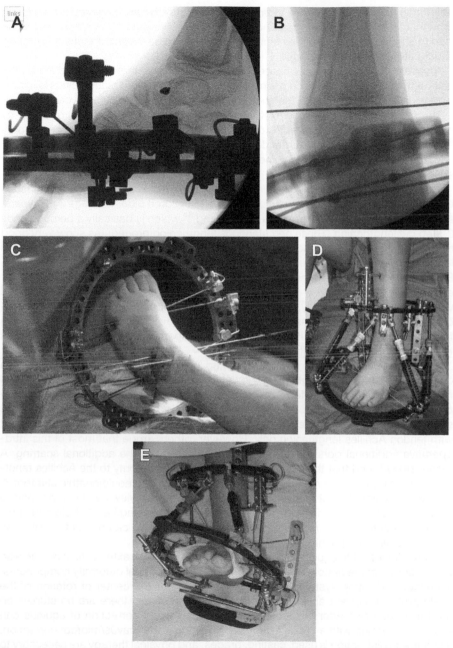

Fig. 1. An olive wire is placed into the neck of the talus from lateral to stabilize the talus during subtalar correction (*A*). The distal tibial epiphysis is protected from epiphysiolysis with a stirrup wire during distraction of the ankle joint necessary for correction of equinus (*B*). The stirrup wire has to be fixed to the proximal ring for the whole time, whereas the talar neck wire is moved from the proximal to the distal ring for correction of equinus (*C*, *D*). For correction of adductus and cavus, the distal ring is cut with a Gigli saw with removal of a piece of the ring lateral and the whole construct is converted into an unconstrained frame (*E*).

tenotomy), with noncompliance to bracing, or as a slow developing recurrence during growth. Especially when the baseline dorsiflexion is less than 10°, growth spurts can lead to shortening of the Achilles tendon. Therefore, home-based stretching exercises should always be recommended.

A severe equinus deformity causes functional limitation that severely disturbs the gait pattern. A very frequent compensation mechanism even in mild equinus is hyperextension of the knee joint at the end of the stance phase in the gait cycle.

The initial equinus component of the clubfoot deformity is usually corrected by percutaneous tenotomy as part of the Ponseti treatment. Various procedures for lengthening of the Achilles tendon in equinus deformity have been described[51] and the biomechanical effects and structures at risk were examined in cadaver specimens.[52,53]

In an early recurrence of equinus in children with clubfoot a repeated percutaneous tendon Achilles lengthening can be performed. In children older than age 3 to 4 years, these authors prefer a Hoke Achilles lengthening,[54] which is basically a percutaneous 3-step cut lengthening. These percutaneous lengthening procedures show very good results in feet not having undergone previous open release surgery or open Achilles lengthening and provide about 10° of dorsiflexion in the typical clubfoot recurrence. Even in feet after open surgery, a percutaneous tenotomy can be performed. However, there is an increased risk of bleeding because structures might have a scarred and variant position. Additionally, massive scarring after open surgery might limit the increase in dorsiflexion. It was suggested that even owing to peritendinous scarring from tenotomy during initial Ponseti treatment, a repeated lengthening of the Achilles tendon can be less successful.[55]

Open Achilles lengthening can be performed in children older than 6 to 8 years or in cases of previous open lengthening. However, physical therapy after cast removal is necessary to minimize scar formation and subsequent loss of motion. The role of the posterior joint capsule in preventing dorsiflexion is still under discussion. Some surgeons state that a posterior release provides additional dorsiflexion compared with tendon Achilles lengthening only. However, others argue that most of this intraoperative additional dorsiflexion is lost later on, owing to the additional scarring. A recent study found that the addition of a posterior capsulotomy to the Achilles tenotomy did not improve the mean dorsiflexion in idiopathic and nonidiopathic clubfoot.[56]

In children older than 2 to 4 years, a lateral ankle mortise view can be performed to analyze the talar dome and predict the result of an Achilles lengthening before the procedure. An anterior subluxation of the talus or flat top talus can prevent dorsiflexion despite Achilles lengthening.

Correction of ankle equinus by soft tissue distraction using external fixation can also be performed alone or combined with correction of additional deformity components. A constrained frame system with hinges positioned at the center of rotation of the ankle joint can correct ankle equinus. Unfortunately, again there are no studies on the recurrence rate after this kind of correction. Gradual correction of equinus can also be performed with a 6-axis fixator in combination with cavus/midfoot correction. If soft tissue distraction is used, casting, braces, and physical therapy are necessary to prevent early recurrence.

As another approach to increase dorsiflexion or prevent equinus, the guided growth concept—commonly used for correction of angular deformities—has been applied to the anterior distal tibia. However, Al-Aubaidi et al[57] reported disappointing results after anterior distal tibial hemiepiphysiodesis in children with fixed recurrent equinus with former clubfoot surgery. The radiographic measurement of the (over)corrected anterior distal tibial angle did not correlate with an increase in clinical ankle range of motion. The authors saw a possible reason in the posterior ankle soft tissue contracture, which was not addressed by this procedure. Anterior subluxation of the talus within the ankle mortise might play an additional role.

In cases with severe flat top talus or incongruent semistiff ankle joints, a supramalleolar equinus correction can be performed. Napiontek and Nazar[58] described tibial osteotomy as a salvage procedure for children with severe clubfeet. The authors stated that the indications for this compensatory procedure are exceptionally rare.[58]

The recent study of Nelman and colleagues[59] reviewed the results of multiplanar supramalleolar osteotomies as a salvage procedure in children with complex rigid foot deformities. Seven of the 18 included patients had severe recurrent clubfoot. Correction of equinus, rotation, and varus was performed with an anterior approach to the distal one-third of the tibia. The age at surgery in patients with clubfoot ranged from 2 to 13 years and the 7 patients with 9 severe clubfeet showed failure of treatment in 4 feet (44%). Failure was defined as recurrence of deformity, nonplantigrade foot at follow-up, or if another supramalleolar osteotomy had to be performed.

Supramalleolar osteotomies for clubfoot should only be performed at the very end of growth, because remaining growth leads to remodeling and thereby recurrence of the equinus. Additionally, massive overcorrection of the anterior distal tibial angle may lead to subluxation of the talus without gaining dorsiflexion and possible early arthrosis owing to cartilage shear forces.

In adolescents and young adults, bony salvage can be performed with external fixation through a supramalleolar correction. With a 6-axis external fixator equinus, varus and rotation can be corrected simultaneously. In the presence of leg length discrepancy, a second proximal tibial osteotomy can be performed for lengthening (**Fig. 2**). Lengthening of the distal tibia should be avoided or kept to a minimum, because this often leads to arthrosis of the ankle joint.

CAVUS

In evaluation of equinus the midfoot equinus (cavus) component has to be considered. Cavus as the residual after treatment of atypical clubfoot can resolve after weight bearing and further growth, and can be observed. In recurrences in patients up to the age of 6 to 8 years, a cavus component can usually be corrected sufficiently with a plantar fasciotomy. The authors prefer a percutaneous approach using an 18-G needle inserted at the insertion of the plantar fascia at the calcaneus. Care must be taken to only section the fascia layers without injuring the plantar nerve. Alternatively, a fascia resection can be performed from a plantar–medial approach. Many authors report plantar fasciotomy combined with external fixation[50] with midfoot osteotomies,[60,61] with calcaneal osteotomy[62] or in correction of neglected clubfoot.[63]

For rigid and fixed cavus, resection of tarsal bones has been described as a salvage procedure. Japas[64] described a tarsal V-osteotomy in neurogenic cavus feet for children older than 6 years. Mubarak and Dimeglio[65] described the excision of the navicular bone through a medial incision combined with a cuboid closing wedge resection to treat pediatric cavovarus deformity. However, resection of tarsal bones further shortens the already short foot, which is not only a cosmetic, but also a shoe-fitting problem. If only some bone is resected but the cavus is still fully corrected acutely, there is the risk of neurovascular complications.

A gradual correction of cavus with an external fixator can be performed.[66–68] This can be achieved with an Ilizarov or with a 6-axis external fixator like the Taylor spatial frame, which also allows to correct pro- and supination and adductus through the same osteotomy. The authors use a Taylor spatial frame in a so-called Butt frame

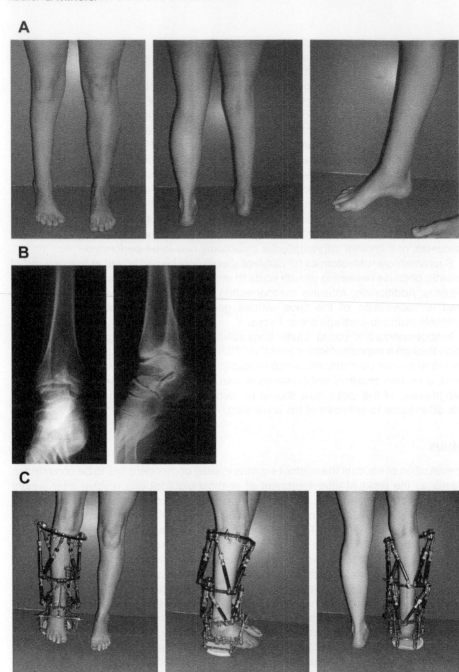

Fig. 2. (*A*) This 16-year-old girl presented with fixed equinus, a pain-free ankle joint, and a leg length discrepancy of 3.3 cm. Further, in-toing with partial compensation through hip rotation and mild heel varus were observed. (*B*) Radiographs revealed a triangular-shaped ankle joint, most likely as the result of the initial surgery. (*C*) A bilevel Taylor spatial frame was applied for lengthening at the proximal osteotomy and equinus, varus, and mild rotational correction through a supramalleolar osteotomy. (*D*) After the operation, a radiographically (*E*) and clinically (*F*) functional foot position was achieved. Only 3 months after frame removal, a good gait pattern was observed (Video 1).

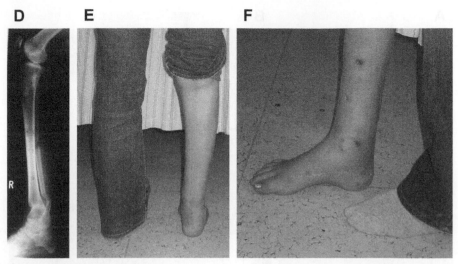

Fig. 2. (*continued*).

(butt joint frame; **Fig. 3**) or Miter frame (miter joint frame; **Fig. 4**A–F) configuration. For selective midfoot/cavus correction, a butt frame construct is sufficient and very powerful. A miter frame construct allows additional equinus correction in the ankle joint. In children older than 6 to 8 years, correction should be performed through a midfoot Gigli saw osteotomy, because soft tissue distraction might lead to recurrence. For gradual cavus and especially cavus and equinus correction, the toes must be transfixed to prevent clawing and contractures of the toes (see **Fig. 4**C, D), a complication commonly described in external fixation for clubfoot.[69–72]

External fixation for cavus and equinus in clubfoot has also been reported in a series of very young patients.[73] Again, with the good results achieved with the Ponseti method, the authors see no indication for external fixation in such young patient groups. The main indications for us to consider external fixation are previously extensively operated feet with massive scarring, critical soft tissues, and extreme deformity.

ADDUCTION

Dynamic forefoot adduction with supination is the main indication for TATT. The use of TATT in the treatment of recurrent clubfoot was first described by Garceau.[74] The technique was modified by Ponseti and implemented as part of treatment for recurrence in the Ponseti method.[75]

Holt and colleagues[76] conducted a 47-year follow-up of recurrent clubfoot treated with TATT. They conclude that TATT is a safe procedure for dynamic relapse without negative effects on long-term foot function. No patient of the TATT group experienced recurrence or additional foot operations at a follow-up of 47 years. Although Holt and colleagues[76] did not have any recurrence in their group of TATT in long term follow-up, other authors observed a second recurrence in 15% to 20% after TATT in other patient series.[20,77] These feet should undergo further examination regarding neuromuscular etiology.

TATT is the first choice for all recurrences where subtalar derotation is corrected or was achieved by casting. Additionally, it can be used in combination with other

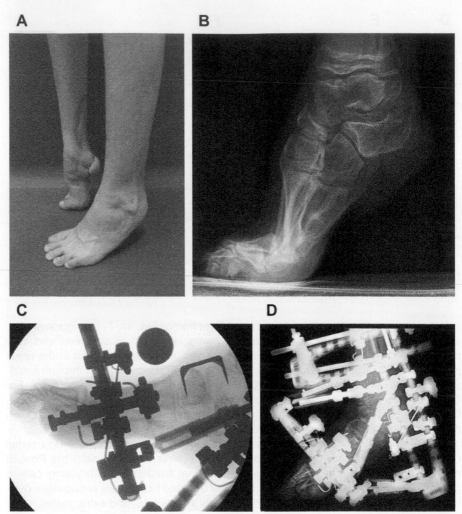

Fig. 3. A 10-year-old boy presented with a non–shoe-able clubfoot on the right side with massive cavus and equinus and a clubfoot with mild equinus that was manageable well in an orthopedic shoe on the left side (*A, B*). The soft tissue situation was critical after previous operations performed elsewhere that resulted in infection, skin necrosis, and the need for plastic surgery (*A*). Intraoperatively, a partial acute correction was performed and temporarily stabilized with a staple while a Taylor spatial frame in a butt frame configuration was applied (*C*). Afterward, a slow gradual correction was performed (*D*). Owing to impending risk of scar breakdown anterior on the dorsum of the foot, the correction was stopped before neutral foot position (*E*). However, the patient was mobilized well with an orthopedic shoe and was very satisfied with the result.

procedures to restore muscle balance and prevent re-recurrence in the treatment of severe recurrent clubfeet.

Although dynamic and flexible forefoot adduction is usually the result of muscle imbalance, fixed forefoot adduction is found more frequently as a residual than recurrent deformity. Residual forefoot adduction may not be a severe problem per se, but it can lead to shoe fitting problems or be one part of a more complex deformity.

E

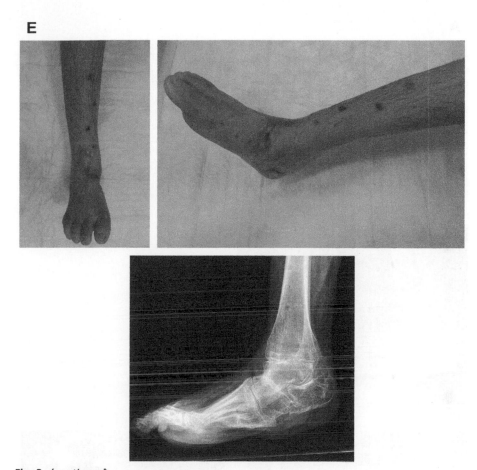

Fig. 3. (*continued*).

McHale and Lenhart[78] reported the combination of a cuboid closing with a cuneiform opening wedge osteotomy in children with clubfoot with residual adductus in the midfoot. As one advantage, they described that it could be used in children too old for release operations but too young for triple arthrodesis.[78] However, from our perspective, these 3 operations target very different deformities and show very different potential of correction.

Clinical and radiographic improvement with lateral column shortening and medial column lengthening sometimes combined with additional procedures has also been described by other authors.[60,61,79] Combinations of closing wedge cuboid and transcuneiform osteotomies in children with residual forefoot adduction 4 to 5 years of age[80] and a combined closing wedge cuboid and opening wedge medial cuneiform with transcuneiform osteotomy in 4 to 9 years old children[81] have also been described.

Most authors report the fixation of midtarsal osteotomies with Kirschner wires.[60,61,78,80,81] For lateral column shortening and medial column lengthening in older children, these authors prefer fixation with a compression staple on the cuboid and a standard staple on the medial cuneiform (**Fig. 5**). Furthermore, adduction can also be corrected as part of a gradual midfoot correction using external fixation.

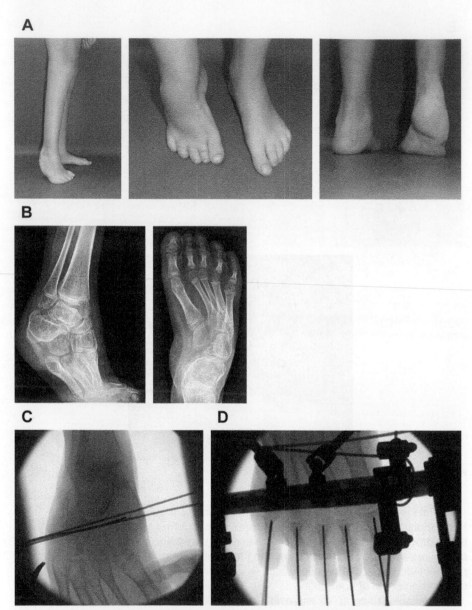

Fig. 4. This girl presented at the age of 8 years after 2 operations and a severe equinus (*A*). Radiographs revealed a massive cavus and ankle equinus (*B*). A midfoot osteotomy between 2 stirrup wires, focusing the distraction forces on the osteotomy, was performed (*C*). Fixation of the toes is necessary in correction of severe equinus and/or cavus to prevent toe contractures (*D*). A small walking platform was attached to the frame to allow for partial weight bearing with crutches (*E*). The midfoot equinus/cavus was corrected through the osteotomy, and a soft tissue distraction was done at the ankle joint to correct equinus (*F*). The radiographs after frame removal showed a very good foot position and the typical osteopenia after 4 months in the frame (*G*). A walking cast was used afterward to consolidate the correction and allow for a gradual increase in weight bearing.

E

F

G

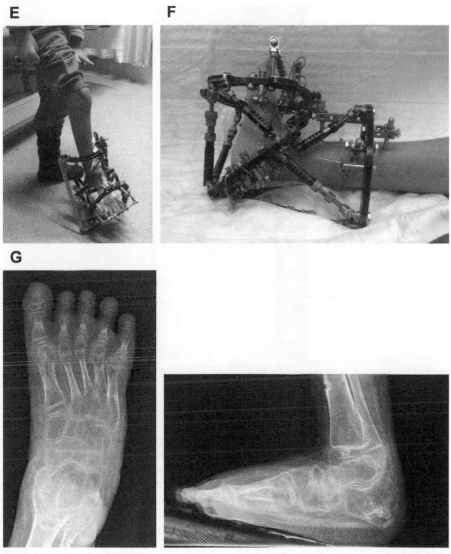

Fig. 4. (continued).

HEEL VARUS

In cases where subtalar derotation is not achieved, heel varus (calcaneal inversion combined with adduction) persists. Many procedures have been introduced to correct heel varus through osteotomies or fusions of the calcaneus. Popular operations were the Dwyer osteotomy or Evans procedure. Dwyer[62] treated relapsed clubfoot with an extraarticular medial opening wedge calcaneus osteotomy at age 2.5 to 3 years. In his opinion and in contrast with the treatment regime of Evans,[82] Dwyer advocated to not excise any bone at the midtarsal or subtalar joints, which would "mutilate and produce permanent stiffness." The Dwyer calcaneal osteotomy was widely used as medial opening wedge osteotomy[62,83–86] or a lateral closing wedge osteotomy.[83,87–90]

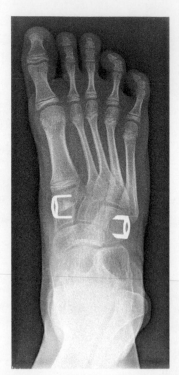

Fig. 5. Correction of isolated but fixed forefoot adduction is rarely necessary, but can be achieved through a medial cuneiform opening wedge and a cuboid closing wedge osteotomy and fixed with stables.

Although medial opening wedge osteotomies showed high rates of wound healing problems, lateral closing wedge osteotomies resulted in decreased foot height.[84]

Evans[82] described an operative procedure for the "unreduced" or relapsed clubfoot at the age of 4 to 5 years to avoid the need of triple arthrodesis. In fixed deformities, he performed a medial and posterior release and a wedge resection at the calcaneocuboid joint. With the shortening of the lateral pillar, the talonavicular dislocation and heel varus should be corrected. A cohort of patients after Evans clubfoot procedures has been reported with a midterm follow-up of 5 years[33] and long-term follow-up of 17 years.[91] Compared with the first evaluation, the rate of excellent functional scores dropped from 85% to 38%. However, no other operations after the Evans procedure were performed during that follow-up and low pain was reported.[91]

Presently, calcaneocuboid fusion without a medial release might rarely be indicated in cases of recurrent syndromic or neurogenic clubfoot. The original Dwyer clubfoot operation is not indicated anymore, but lateralizing calcaneal osteotomies can be performed in adolescents and young adult patients for the correction of heel varus. This lateral slide osteotomy can be performed as a reversed Koutsogiannis osteotomy described for the correction of valgus heel deformities in its original form.[92,93] In very contracted and scarred feet where the slide is limited, it can be combined with the resection of small lateral wedge (mini-Dwyer). If heel varus is corrected in the presence of forefoot pronation with a plantar flexed first metatarsal an elevation osteotomy of the metatarsal should be added (**Fig. 6**). The original Dwyer and Evans procedures are almost obsolete, especially in the age groups for which they were originally described.

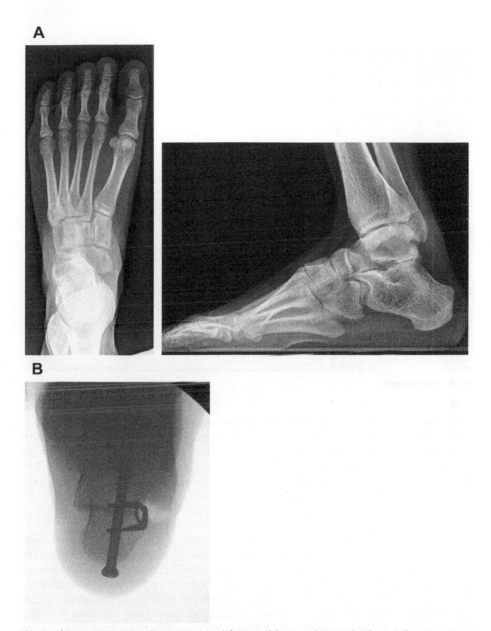

Fig. 6. This young adult who was treated for a mild to moderate clubfoot deformity at our institution before the introduction of the Ponseti method presented with a mild recurrence/residual. Owing to the incomplete subtalar derotation, the heel was in varus and the first ray was plantar flexed (*A*). She complained of a hindfoot instability and pain and pressure under the first metatarsal head. A calcaneal lateralizing osteotomy (*B*) combined with an elevation of the first metatarsal corrected her deformity and alleviated the symptoms (*C*).

In children with hindfoot varus, additional midfoot deformities and pain, triple arthrodesis might be indicated, especially in severe recurrence in neurogenic and syndromic clubfoot. Triple arthrodesis is successfully used in adults with hindfoot deformities to relieve pain and improve functional deficits.[94] It was recognized early that in

C

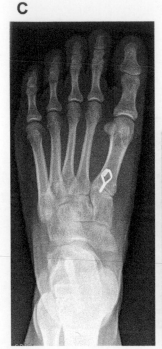

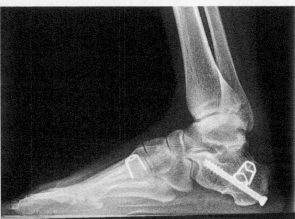

Fig. 6. (*continued*).

small children 6 or 7 years of age the thick layer of cartilage makes it hard to achieve bony contact for arthrodesis. After the age of 10 years, the cartilage gets thinner with more success of arthrodesis.[95] Therefore, triple arthrodesis was recommended for children with severe recurrent clubfoot deformity older than 8 to 10 years.[33,35,90] Penny[63] reported a modified Lambrinudi triple arthrodesis with a high potential to correct even most severe clubfoot deformities. He has successfully used this modified technique to treat stiff neglected clubfoot in patients from age 6 in the context of developing nations.

Kuhns and colleagues[96] compared the growth rates of children treated with triple arthrodesis. Skeletally immature children younger than 10 years showed no significant growth changes compared with skeletal mature children older than 10 years. However high rates of residual deformity in children with clubfoot treated with triple arthrodesis[97,98] and severe complications such as wound infections, pseudoarthrosis, osteomyelitis, talus necrosis, and even amputation have been reported.[97] Triple arthrodesis has without question a high power in correction of hindfoot and midfoot deformities. The indication in children with clubfoot is extremely rare. It should be held back as a last resort or for adult patients with symptomatic osteoarthritic changes.

SUMMARY

Strict adherence to the Ponseti treatment protocol, ensuring and enforcing brace compliance, frequent follow-up, and early treatment of recurrence prevents severe recurrence and the need for invasive operative procedures. Rarely are we faced with previously operated, neurogenic, or syndromic clubfoot that cannot be sufficiently corrected with the Ponseti method. For those feet, we have to find the smallest procedure that durably increases function, yet loses as little joint mobility as possible. Indicating the right treatment and surgical procedure is crucial and should always be guided by individual patient needs and functional considerations. A countless number of procedures and combinations of those have been reported with most of them obsolete or outdated. There is a current trend toward external fixation for very stiff clubfoot with severe deformity and/or critical skin conditions because it allows for gradual correction and minimal invasive osteotomies. However, the long-term functional outcomes of this small and heterogenic patient population treated with various external fixation techniques are rarely reported.

Understanding the pathoanatomy and its implication on treatment options is important for the successful treatment of severe recurrent clubfoot. A comprehensive clinical evaluation of the different components of clubfoot helps in selecting the adequate procedures. The individual needs and especially the social and psychological factors influencing treatment and the impact of treatment on the child have to be considered. With increasing dissemination and improved understanding of the Ponseti method a further reduction in the frequency of severe recurrent clubfoot can be hoped for and expected.

SUPPLEMENTARY DATA

Supplementary data related to this article can be found online at http://dx.doi.org/10.1016/j.fcl.2015.07.002.

REFERENCES

1. Dobbs MB, Morcuende JA, Gurnett CA, et al. Treatment of idiopathic clubfoot: an historical review. Iowa Orthop J 2000;20:59–64.
2. McKay DW. New concept of and approach to clubfoot treatment: section II–correction of the clubfoot. J Pediatr Orthop 1983;3(1):10–21.
3. Simons GW. Complete subtalar release in club feet. Part I–A preliminary report. J Bone Joint Surg Am 1985;67(7):1044–55.
4. Turco VJ. Surgical correction of the resistant club foot. One-stage posteromedial release with internal fixation: a preliminary report. J Bone Joint Surg Am 1971; 53(3):477–97.
5. Aronson J, Puskarich CL. Deformity and disability from treated clubfoot. J Pediatr Orthop 1990;10(1):109–19.
6. Dobbs MB, Nunley R, Schoenecker PL. Long-term follow-up of patients with clubfeet treated with extensive soft-tissue release. J Bone Joint Surg Am 2006;88(5): 986–96.
7. Green AD, Lloyd-Roberts GC. The results of early posterior release in resistant club feet. A long-term review. J Bone Joint Surg Br 1985;67(4):588–93.
8. Atar D, Lehman WB, Grant AD. Complications in clubfoot surgery. Orthop Rev 1991;20(3):233–9.
9. Cooper DM, Dietz FR. Treatment of idiopathic clubfoot. A thirty-year follow-up note. J Bone Joint Surg Am 1995;77(10):1477–89.
10. Morcuende JA, Dolan LA, Dietz FR, et al. Radical reduction in the rate of extensive corrective surgery for clubfoot using the Ponseti method. Pediatrics 2004; 113(2):376–80.
11. Ponseti IV, Smoley EN. The classic: Congenital club foot: The results of treatment. 1963. Clin Orthop Relat Res 2009;467(5):1133–45.

12. Smith PA, Kuo KN, Graf AN, et al. Long-term results of comprehensive clubfoot release versus the Ponseti method: Which is better? Clin Orthop Relat Res 2014;472(4):1281–90.
13. Shabtai L, Specht SC, Herzenberg JE. Worldwide spread of the Ponseti method for clubfoot. World J Orthop 2014;5(5):585–90.
14. Radler C, Mindler GT, Riedl K, et al. Midterm results of the Ponseti method in the treatment of congenital clubfoot. Int Orthop 2013;37(9):1827–31.
15. Mindler GT, Kranzl A, Lipkowski CAM, et al. Results of Gait Analysis Including the Oxford Foot Model in Children with Clubfoot Treated with the Ponseti Method. J Bone Joint Surg Am 2014;96(19):1593–9.
16. Zionts LE, Zhao G, Hitchcock K, et al. Has the rate of extensive surgery to treat idiopathic clubfoot declined in the United States? J Bone Joint Surg Am 2010; 92(4):882–9.
17. Garg S, Dobbs MB. Use of the Ponseti method for recurrent clubfoot following posteromedial release. Indian J Orthop 2008;42(1):68–72.
18. Nogueira MP, Ey Batlle AM, Alves CG. Is it possible to treat recurrent clubfoot with the Ponseti technique after posteromedial release? A preliminary study. Clin Orthop Relat Res 2009;467(5):1298–305.
19. Lovell ME, Morcuende JA. Neuromuscular disease as the cause of late clubfoot relapses: report of 4 cases. Iowa Orthop J 2007;27:82–4.
20. Masrouha KZ, Morcuende JA. Relapse after tibialis anterior tendon transfer in idio-pathic clubfoot treated by the Ponseti method. J Pediatr Orthop 2012;32(1):81–4.
21. Moon DK, Gurnett CA, Aferol H, et al. Soft-tissue abnormalities associated with treatment-resistant and treatment-responsive clubfoot: findings of MRI analysis. J Bone Joint Surg Am 2014;96(15):1249–56.
22. Khan SA, Kumar A. Ponseti's manipulation in neglected clubfoot in children more than 7 years of age: a prospective evaluation of 25 feet with long-term follow-up. J Pediatr Orthop B 2010;19(5):385–9.
23. Lourenço AF, Morcuende JA. Correction of neglected idiopathic club foot by the Ponseti method. J Bone Joint Surg Br 2007;89(3):378–81.
24. Spiegel DA, Shrestha OP, Sitoula P, et al. Ponseti method for untreated idiopathic clubfeet in Nepalese patients from 1 to 6 years of age. Clin Orthop Relat Res 2009;467(5):1164–70.
25. Shaheen S, Jaiballa H, Pirani S. Interobserver reliability in Pirani clubfoot severity scoring between a paediatric orthopaedic surgeon and a physiotherapy assis-tant. J Pediatr Orthop B 2012;21(4):366–8.
26. Diméglio A, Bensahel H, Souchet P, et al. Classification of clubfoot. J Pediatr Orthop B 1995;4(2):129–36.
27. Bensahel H, Dimeglio A, Souchet P. Final evaluation of clubfoot. J Pediatr Orthop B 1995;4(2):137–41.
28. Bhaskar A, Patni P. Classification of relapse pattern in clubfoot treated with Pon-seti technique. Indian J Orthop 2013;47(4):370–6.
29. Farsetti P, Dragoni M, Ippolito E. Tibiofibular torsion in congenital clubfoot. J Pediatr Orthop B 2012;21(1):47–51.
30. Sankar WN, Rethlefsen SA, Weiss J, et al. The recurrent clubfoot: Can gait anal-ysis help us make better preoperative decisions? Clin Orthop Relat Res 2009; 467(5):1214–22.
31. Schleicher I, Lappas K, Klein H, et al. Follow up of complete subtalar release for clubfoot-Evolution of different scores. Foot Ankle Surg 2012;18(1):55–61.
32. Lehman WB, Atar D, Grant AD, et al. Re-do clubfoot: surgical approach and long-term results. Bull N Y Acad Med 1990;66(6):601–17.

33. Lehman WB, Atar D, Bash J, et al. Results of complete soft tissue clubfoot release combined with calcaneocuboid fusion in the 4-year to 8-year age group following failed clubfoot release. J Pediatr Orthop B 1999;8(3):181–6.
34. Turco VJ. Resistant congenital club foot–one-stage posteromedial release with internal fixation. A follow-up report of a fifteen-year experience. J Bone Joint Surg Am 1979;61(6A):805–14.
35. Ettl V, Kirschner S, Krauspe R, et al. Midterm results following revision surgery in clubfeet. Int Orthop 2009;33(2):515–20.
36. Kamath BJ, Bhardwaj P. Local flap coverage following posteromedial release in clubfoot surgery in older children. Int Orthop 2005;29(1):39–41.
37. Haasbeek JF, Zuker RM, Wright JG. Free gracilis muscle transfer for coverage of severe foot deformities. J Pediatr Orthop 1995;15(5):608–12.
38. Khan MA, Chinoy MA. Treatment of severe and neglected clubfoot with a double zigzag incision: outcome of 21 feet in 15 patients followed up Between 1 and 5 years. J Foot Ankle Surg 2006;45(3):177–81.
39. Burns JK, Sullivan R. Correction of severe residual clubfoot deformity in adolescents with the Ilizarov technique. Foot Ankle Clin 2004;9(3):571–82.
40. El-Mowafi H, El-Alfy B, Refai M. Functional outcome of salvage of residual and recurrent deformities of clubfoot with Ilizarov technique. Foot Ankle Surg 2009; 15(1):3–6.
41. Ferreira RC, Costa MT. Recurrent clubfoot-approach and treatment with external fixation. Foot Ankle Clin 2009;14(3):435–45.
42. Grant AD, Atar D, Lehman WB. The Ilizarov technique in correction of complex foot deformities. Clin Orthop Relat Res 1992;(280):94–103.
43. Grill F, Franke J. The Ilizarov distractor for the correction of relapsed or neglected clubfoot. J Bone Joint Surg Br 1987;69(4):593–7.
44. Kocaoğlu M, Eralp L, Atalar AC, et al. Correction of complex foot deformities using the Ilizarov external fixator. J Foot Ankle Surg 2002;41(1):30–9.
45. Tripathy SK, Saini R, Sudes P, et al. Application of the Ponseti principle for deformity correction in neglected and relapsed clubfoot using the Ilizarov fixator. J Pediatr Orthop B 2011;20(1):26–32.
46. Lamm BM, Standard SC, Galley IJ, et al. External fixation for the foot and ankle in children. Clin Podiatr Med Surg 2006;23(1):137–66.
47. Ganger R, Radler C, Handlbauer A, et al. External fixation in clubfoot treatment – a review of the literature. J Pediatr Orthop B 2012;21(1):52–8.
48. Choi IH, Yang MS, Chung CY, et al. The treatment of recurrent arthrogrypotic club foot in children by the Ilizarov method. A preliminary report. J Bone Joint Surg Br 2001;83(5):731–7.
49. El Barbary H, Abdel Ghani H, Hegazy M. Correction of relapsed or neglected clubfoot using a simple Ilizarov frame. Int Orthop 2004;28(3):183–6.
50. Ferreira RC, Costa MT, Frizzo GG, et al. Correction of severe recurrent clubfoot using a simplified setting of the Ilizarov device. Foot Ankle Int 2007;28(5): 557–68.
51. Dietz FR, Albright JC, Dolan L. Medium-term follow-up of Achilles tendon lengthening in the treatment of ankle equinus in cerebral palsy. Iowa Orthop J 2006;26: 27–32.
52. Firth GB, McMullan M, Chin T, et al. Lengthening of the gastrocnemius-soleus complex: an anatomical and biomechanical study in human cadavers. J Bone Joint Surg Am 2013;95(16):1489–96.
53. Salamon ML, Pinney SJ, Van Bergeyk A, et al. Surgical anatomy and accuracy of percutaneous Achilles tendon lengthening. Foot Ankle Int 2006;27(6):411–3.

54. Hoke M. An operation for stabilizing paralytic feet. J Orthop Surg 1921;3(10): 494–507.
55. Chu A, Lehman WB. Persistent clubfoot deformity following treatment by the Ponseti method. J Pediatr Orthop B 2012;21(1):40–6.
56. Grigoriou E, Abol Oyoun N, Kushare I, et al. Comparative results of percutaneous Achilles tenotomy to combined open Achilles tenotomy with posterior capsulotomy in the correction of equinus deformity in congenital talipes equinovarus. Int Orthop 2015;39(4):721–5.
57. Al-Aubaidi Z, Lundgaard B, Pedersen NW. Anterior distal tibial epiphysiodesis for the treatment of recurrent equinus deformity after surgical treatment of clubfeet. J Pediatr Orthop 2011;31(6):716–20.
58. Napiontek M, Nazar J. Tibial osteotomy as a salvage procedure in the treatment of congenital talipes equinovarus. J Pediatr Orthop 1994;14(6):763–7.
59. Nelman K, Weiner DS, Morscher MA, et al. Multiplanar supramalleolar osteotomy in the management of complex rigid foot deformities in children. J Child Orthop 2009;3(1):39–46.
60. Loza ME, Bishay SN, El-Barbary HM, et al. Double column osteotomy for correction of residual adduction deformity in idiopathic clubfoot. Ann R Coll Surg Engl 2010;92(8):673–9.
61. Schaefer D, Hefti F. Combined cuboid/cuneiform osteotomy for correction of residual adductus deformity in idiopathic and secondary club feet. J Bone Joint Surg Br 2000;82(6):881–4.
62. Dwyer FC. Treatment of the relapsed club foot. Proc R Soc Med 1968;61(8):783.
63. Penny JN. The Neglected Clubfoot. Tech Orthop 2005;20(2):153–66.
64. Japas LM. Surgical treatment of pes cavus by tarsal V-osteotomy. Preliminary report. J Bone Joint Surg Am 1968;50(5):927–44.
65. Mubarak SJ, Dimeglio A. Navicular excision and cuboid closing wedge for severe cavovarus foot deformities: a salvage procedure. J Pediatr Orthop 2011;31(5): 551–6.
66. Eidelman M, Katzman A. Treatment of complex foot deformities in children with the Taylor spatial frame. Orthopedics 2008;31(10). pii: orthosupersite.com/view.asp?rID=31514.
67. Eidelman M, Keren Y, Katzman A. Correction of residual clubfoot deformities in older children using the Taylor spatial butt frame and midfoot Gigli saw osteotomy. J Pediatr Orthop 2012;32(5):527–33.
68. Paley D, Lamm BM. Correction of the cavus foot using external fixation. Foot Ankle Clin 2004;9(3):611–24.
69. de la Huerta F. Correction of the neglected clubfoot by the Ilizarov method. Clin Orthop Relat Res 1994;(301):89–93.
70. Gupta P, Bither N. Ilizarov in relapsed clubfoot: a necessary evil? J Pediatr Orthop B 2013;22(6):589–94.
71. Khanfour AA. Ilizarov techniques with limited adjunctive surgical procedures for the treatment of preadolescent recurrent or neglected clubfeet. J Pediatr Orthop B 2013;22(3):240–8.
72. Refai MA, Song SH, Song HR. Does short-term application of an Ilizarov frame with transfixion pins correct relapsed clubfoot in children? Clin Orthop Relat Res 2012;470(7):1992–9.
73. Suresh S, Ahmed A, Sharma VK. Role of Joshi's external stabilisation system fixator in the management of idiopathic clubfoot. J Orthop Surg (Hong Kong) 2003; 11(2):194–201.

74. Garceau GJ. Anterior tibial tendon transfer for recurrent clubfoot. Clin Orthop Relat Res 1972;84:61–5.
75. Ponseti IV. Congenital clubfoot: fundamentals of treatment. New York: Oxford University Press; 1996. p. 84.
76. Holt JB, Oji DE, Yack HJ, et al. Long-term results of tibialis anterior tendon transfer for relapsed idiopathic clubfoot treated with the Ponseti method: a follow-up of thirty-seven to fifty-five years. J Bone Joint Surg Am 2015;97(1):47–55.
77. Luckett MR, Hosseinzadeh P, Ashley PA, et al. Factors predictive of second recurrence in clubfeet treated by Ponseti casting. J Pediatr Orthop 2015;35(3): 303–6.
78. McHale KA, Lenhart MK. Treatment of residual clubfoot deformity–the "bean-shaped" foot–by opening wedge medial cuneiform osteotomy and closing wedge cuboid osteotomy. Clinical review and cadaver correlations. J Pediatr Orthop 1991;11(3):374–81.
79. Lourenco AF, Dias LS, Zoellick DM, et al. Treatment of residual adduction deformity in clubfoot: the double osteotomy. J Pediatr Orthop 2001;21(6):713–8.
80. Mahadev A, Munajat I, Mansor A, et al. Combined lateral and transcuneiform without medial osteotomy for residual clubfoot for children. Clin Orthop Relat Res 2009;467(5):1319–25.
81. Elgeidi A, Abulsaad M. Combined double tarsal wedge osteotomy and transcuneiform osteotomy for correction of resistant clubfoot deformity (the "bean-shaped" foot). J Child Orthop 2014;8(5):399–404.
82. Evans D. Treatment of the unreduced or 'relapsed' club foot in older children. Proc R Soc Med 1968;61(8):782–3.
83. Barenfeld PA, Weseley MS, Munters M. Dwyer calcaneal osteotomy. Clin Orthop Relat Res 1967;53:147–53.
84. Kumar PN, Laing PW, Klenerman L. Medial calcaneal osteotomy for relapsed equinovarus deformity. Long-term study of the results of Frederick Dwyer. J Bone Joint Surg Br 1993;75(6):967–71.
85. Lundberg BJ. Early Dwyer operation in talipes equinovarus. Clin Orthop Relat Res 1981;(154):223–7.
86. Weseley MS, Barenfeld PA. Mechanism of the Dwyer calcaneal osteotomy. Clin Orthop Relat Res 1970;70:137–40.
87. Dwyer FC. Osteotomy of the calcaneum for pes cavus. J Bone Joint Surg Br 1959;41-B(1):80–6.
88. Fisher RL, Shaffer SR. An evaluation of calcaneal osteotomy in congenital clubfoot and other disorders. Clin Orthop Relat Res 1970;70:141–7.
89. Krackow KA, Hales D, Jones L. Preoperative planning and surgical technique for performing a Dwyer calcaneal osteotomy. J Pediatr Orthop 1985;5(2):214–8.
90. Weseley MS, Barenfeld PA. Operative treatment of congenital clubfoot. Clin Orthop Relat Res 1968;59:161–5.
91. Chu A, Chaudhry S, Sala DA, et al. Calcaneocuboid arthrodesis for recurrent clubfeet: What is the outcome at 17-year follow-up? J Child Orthop 2014;8(1): 43–8.
92. Koutsogiannis E. Treatment of mobile flat foot by displacement osteotomy of the calcaneus. J Bone Joint Surg Br 1971;53(1):96–100.
93. Rathjen KE, Mubarak SJ. Calcaneal-cuboid-cuneiform osteotomy for the correction of valgus foot deformities in children. J Pediatr Orthop 1998;18(6):775–82.
94. Pell RF 4th, Myerson MS, Schon LC. Clinical outcome after primary triple arthrodesis. J Bone Joint Surg Am 2000;82(1):47–57.

95. Ryerson EW. Arthrodesing operations on the feet: Edwin W. Ryerson MD (1872-1961). The 1st president of the AAOS 1932. Clin Orthop Relat Res 2008; 466(1):5–14.
96. Kuhns CA, Zeegen EN, Kono M, et al. Growth rates in skeletally immature feet after triple arthrodesis. J Pediatr Orthop 2003;23(4):488–92.
97. Angus PD, Cowell HR. Triple arthrodesis. A critical long-term review. J Bone Joint Surg Br 1986;68(2):260–5.
98. Seitz DG, Carpenter EB. Triple arthrodesis in children: a ten-year review. South Med J 1974;67(12):1420–4.

Evaluation and Surgical Management of the Overcorrected Clubfoot Deformity in the Adult Patient

Dawid Burger, MD, Amiethab Aiyer, MD*, Mark S. Myerson, MD

KEYWORDS

- Clubfoot • Overcorrection • Dorsal bunion • Flattop talus
- Dorsal navicular subluxation

KEY POINTS

- The overcorrected clubfoot is a complication seen as the result of attempts to surgical address previously existing clubfoot deformity.
- Despite the infrequency with which the posteromedial release is performed today, this entity will present occasionally to the orthopedic foot and ankle surgeon.
- A sound understanding of the underlying muscle imbalance is essential when addressing the resulting deformities.
- The surgical aim is to provide the patient with a pain-free, stable, and plantigrade foot that is in neutral alignment.

INTRODUCTION

The overcorrected clubfoot represents a spectrum of deformity that follows a fairly consistent pattern. It may remain asymptomatic for years and the patient often presents only in adulthood. Historically, surgical correction obtained by extensive soft tissue release was the standard of care; the posteromedial release being the mainstay of treatment. Long-term outcomes of clubfoot patients treated with a posteromedial release have demonstrated significant stiffness and arthritis of the foot with revision surgery to address undercorrection or overcorrection a frequent finding.[1]

In comparison, modern treatment of clubfoot is by Ponseti casting, which has been shown to have good long term outcomes.[2–5] Most patients are successfully treated nonoperatively with Ponseti casting[6] and only in a minority of these patients, surgical

The authors have nothing to disclose.
Department of Orthopaedic Surgery, Institute for Foot & Ankle Reconstruction, Mercy Hospital, Mercy Medical Center, 301 St Paul Place, Baltimore, MD 21202, USA
* Corresponding author. Institute for Foot & Ankle Reconstruction, 301 St Paul Place, Baltimore, MD 21202.
E-mail address: tabsaiyer@gmail.com

intervention may be used to augment correction or address recurrent deformity. However, the more traditional posteromedial release is still performed for primary correction in some centers and more commonly for the management of the resistant or recurrent clubfoot. The outcome of treatment, whether nonoperative or operative, seems to be related in some degree to the etiology, and this should be taken into consideration when managing nonidiopathic clubfoot.[7,8]

PRESENTATION
History

Overcorrection occurs almost exclusively in patients who have had prior surgery, usually in the form of a posteromedial release, completed at around 2 years of age. It is not uncommon for many patients to have had additional surgery to either correct a residual deformity or to address overcorrection. There is another spectrum of problems that we treat, where patients have been quite stable for decades but where an anterior ankle cheilectomy is performed for impingement. Decompression of the anterior tibia exposes the underlying abnormal ankle motion secondary to a structurally abnormal flat top talus and, instead of providing pain relief, the cheilectomy leads to an exacerbation of the underlying ankle arthritis.

Patients with an overcorrected clubfoot often present much later in life. They typically give a history of managing for several years with few symptoms, despite the presence of deformity. The onset of acute symptoms or the deterioration of preexisting symptomatology is typically related to minor trauma, such as a sprain of the foot. During early adulthood, the complaints center mostly around the often marked deformity and stiffness that limits activity. These factors lead to discomfort and difficulties with shoe wear. Degenerative joint disease is often seen later in adulthood and is associated with a prior history of good function followed by the insidious onset of progressive pain.

Examination

Physical examination should begin with observation of the gait cycle, the posture of the foot during stance, and while performing a heel rise, if possible. Careful assessment of hindfoot alignment is necessary and its relation with the fore foot should be established.

The authors commonly observe weakness when performing a heel rise indicating a weak or nonfunctioning posterior tibial tendon. When performing a heel rise, the hindfoot does not swing into varus, but may correct only to the midline or stay in fixed valgus, indicating a rigid deformity. To assess for forefoot supination, the ankle is held in a neutral position and the hindfoot alignment corrected while observing the posture of the forefoot. Fixed supination of the forefoot is often seen in the setting of pes planus, and this finding is worse with more flexibility of the hindfoot. With significant hindfoot valgus, tenderness at the tip of the fibula or over the peroneal tendons is the result of calcaneofibular impingement. The navicular is frequently prominent dorsomedially and subluxated from a normal position at the talonavicular and naviculocuneiform joints where arthritis may be present. Tenderness over the anterior aspect of the ankle joint especially in dorsiflexion is caused by anterior ankle impingement.

The ankle, subtalar, and Chopart's joints should be evaluated for mobility and signs of arthritis. It may be difficult to accurately identify the symptomatic joint when all the joints of the hindfoot and ankle radiographically seem to be involved in the process. Selective intraarticular injection using 1% lidocaine under fluoroscopic guidance may help to differentiate between these potential sources of pain. Forefoot deformity is often marked by an elevated first ray with a dorsal bunion of varying prominence. In these feet, hallux metatarsophalangeal (MP) joint dorsiflexion is absent owing to a contracture of the flexor hallucis brevis (FHB). As the first metatarsal moves into more dorsiflexion, the FHB contracts pulling the hallux into even more plantar flexion. This position of the hallux now pushes up on the first metatarsal, which in turn causes more elevation of the first ray until there is a fixed flexion contracture of the hallux with compensatory hyperextension of the hallux interphalangeal joint.

Examination of the strength of the muscles is a good way to understand the underlying dynamic imbalance that is taking place. This evaluation will allow the treating surgeon to better understand the cause of the deformity. Plantar flexion is almost always weak with little excursion of the Achilles tendon owing to the abnormal gastrocnemius/soleus muscle complex and scarring from prior lengthenings of the Achilles tendon. Peroneal muscle weakness seems to be part of the pathology leading to clubfoot, although the reason for this remains uncertain.[9] Scarring of the peroneal tendons is often the result of subfibular impingement or a previous posterolateral release. The anterior tibial tendon remains normal and, therefore, relatively strong compared with its antagonist, the peroneus longus. The imbalance eventually causes an elevation of the medial column often with a varying degree of a dorsal bunion present. The evolution of this is discussed elsewhere in this article. Patients can present with isolated deformities but more often with multiple complaints or deformities.

Nonoperative treatment

Nonoperative treatment options need to be considered before embarking on surgery. These measures can help the patient to overcome a temporary exacerbation of their symptoms and it may enable some to cope without surgery. The use of a custom orthotic often proves to be the most useful and typically consists of a semirigid orthotic support with a medial heel wedge and a post under the first metatarsal to support the elevatus. This support counters the hindfoot valgus and provides support for the resulting elevation in the medial arch. In cases where the symptoms results from painful motion in a degenerative ankle, pain can be controlled with custom bracing such as an Arizona brace or ankle foot orthosis.

MANAGEMENT OF SPECIFIC DEFORMITIES
Hindfoot Valgus

Several factors play a part in this deformity, which is among the most common features of overcorrection[10] (**Fig. 1**). Release of the subtalar joint with transection of

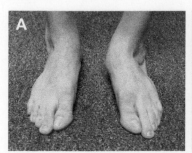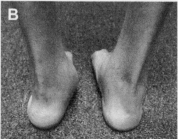

Fig. 1. (*A*, *B*) A 23-year-old patient with an overcorrected left club foot after surgery in childhood. The patient presented with a valgus deformity of the left hindfoot, a symptomatic dorsal bunion, and a painfully subluxated talonavicular joint.

the interosseous talocalcaneal ligament can lead to subtalar instability with lateral translation of the calcaneus relative to the talus and valgus malalignment. Internal fixation by pinning of the subtalar and talonavicular joint after release decrease the risk of overcorrection.[11,12] Intuitively, one tends to attribute the hindfoot valgus to overzealous release of the medial structures, the posterior tibial muscle and talocalcaneal interosseous ligament.[13] However, another likely cause could be the insufficient release of the calcaneofibular ligament lateral, which was shown by Ponseti to be thickened and shortened in the recurrent clubfoot.[14,15] This results in tethering of the foot at the posterolateral corner and, as the foot is dorsiflexed, the subtalar joint is pulled into valgus. With the hindfoot in valgus, the ankle does not function normally. Insertion of the Achilles tendon shifts to a position lateral to the axis of the ankle and subtalar joint and weakens its plantar flexion power. This converts the Achilles tendon into a deforming force that exerts a valgus moment onto the hindfoot that perpetuates the deformity.

The goal of reconstruction is to obtain realignment of the hindfoot by addressing the deformity as close as possible to its apex. It is therefore important to discern ankle valgus from subtalar joint valgus (Fig. 2). In the overcorrected clubfoot, ankle joint valgus often presents with associated calcaneofibular and anterior ankle impingement. In these cases, realignment should be performed with a supramalleolar closing wedge osteotomy.

If ankle joint alignment is normal, the algorithm focuses on the subtalar joint. When considering the subtalar joint the factors taken into consideration are (1) the severity of the deformity, (2) tenderness at the sinus tarsi, (3) the relative flexibility or rigidity of the subtalar joint, and (4) radiographic signs of joint degeneration. In less severe deformities without signs of joint pain, the authors prefer to perform a medial displacement osteotomy of the calcaneus (Fig. 3). If the deformity is severe or significant joint degeneration is present, the authors tend to perform an arthrodesis of the subtalar joint. Realignment can be difficult because the hindfoot may be in severe valgus. Correction of the valgus with an arthrodesis inevitably leads to a large lateral defect that is filled with generous amounts of bone graft. This situation, however, presents a difficulty with respect to decision making of placement of the incision for the arthrodesis. If there is significant valgus deformity, a laterally based incision will not close if the valgus is corrected, and less so if bone graft is used to elevate or change the position of the hindfoot. For this reason, the authors prefer to use a medial approach to correct the subtalar joint when marked hindfoot valgus is present. The same concept applies to correction of deformity when a triple arthrodesis is planned, when we will use a medial approach to the triple arthrodesis (see references for medial triple, Myerson, etc).

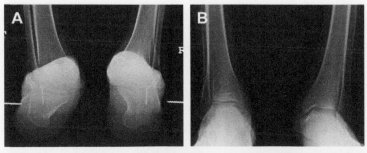

Fig. 2. (A, B) Hindfoot alignment radiographs demonstrates the valgus deformity in the left hindfoot. A weight bearing anterior posterior radiograph of the ankle excludes a valgus deformity at the level of the left ankle joint.

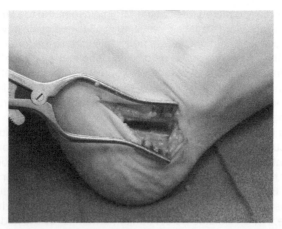

Fig. 3. Intraoperative view of the medializing calcaneal osteotomy performed via a lateral approach to address the hindfoot valgus.

A valgus deformity may be present at both levels and the hindfoot should be evaluated carefully for residual valgus after correction of ankle valgus. When present, consideration should be given for the need of a medializing calcaneal osteotomy. In addition to the subtalar joint, the status of the talonavicular joint should be assessed, which in our experience is more commonly involved in the deformity, necessitating a triple arthrodesis.

Dorsal Bunion

When dealing with the dorsal bunion, it is important to recognize the muscular imbalance created by the relatively normal, and therefore strong, anterior tibial tendon overpowering a weak peroneus longus. This results in an elevation of the first ray and supination of the forefoot (**Fig. 4**). The weak plantar flexion power of the abnormal gastrocnemius–soleus is compensated for by plantar flexion of the hallux MP joint using the secondary plantar flexors such as the FHB. Over time, a functional contracture of the FHB develops. During ambulation, the plantarflexed hallux and proximal

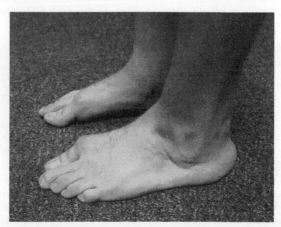

Fig. 4. Bilateral symptomatic dorsal bunions. Note the elevated first metatarsal and contracted flexor hallucis brevis.

phalanx exert a dorsally directed force at the MP joint when the toe strikes the ground, forcing the first ray into more elevation, resulting in a vicious cycle of worsening deformity[16] (**Fig. 5**). With cast treatment, care is taken to supinate the forefoot because pronation increases the underlying cavus deformity. Despite the correct treatment, some patients treated in a cast may have continued supination of the forefoot as well as a dorsal bunion. This muscular imbalance is therefore also seen in feet treated with the Ponseti method at times, necessitating a transfer of the anterior tibial tendon lateral to balance its supination force.[17]

Correction of a dorsal bunion in the setting of an overcorrected clubfoot fails if the underlying muscular imbalance is not corrected and we, therefore, start with a transfer of the anterior tibial tendon. The entire anterior tibial tendon is released at the beginning of the procedure and transferred only once the other corrections are completed (**Fig. 6**). This sequence gives a much better appreciation and feel for the balance of the foot, which will dictate how far laterally in the midfoot the transfer needs to be done. For an isolated dorsal bunion, a transfer to the middle cuneiform is usually sufficient to restore balance. By removing the anterior tibial tendon as a deforming force while maintaining adequate dorsiflexion power, the muscle imbalance is corrected.

The question then becomes whether to fuse the first metatarsocuneiform joint or to perform an osteotomy of the metatarsal. It is the senior author's experience that the rigidity of the deformity is usually of such severity that full correction is impossible with an osteotomy. The authors therefore perform a fusion of the metatarsocuneiform joint in plantar flexion by removing a plantar-based wedge at the metatarsocuneiform joint. This technique allows for some shortening of the metatarsal with relaxation of the FHB and improved dorsiflexion of the first MP joint. Closing the plantar-based wedge usually requires the forceful dorsiflexion of the hallux MP joint to generate enough pressure. Although the force on the hallux is maintained, the saw blade is introduced repeatedly into the metatarsocuneiform joint along the plantar surface to gradually decompress and plantar flex the arthrodesis. The authors do not recommend a dorsal opening wedge osteotomy of the first metatarsal, because this is usually not powerful enough and the further lengthening of the metatarsal causes even more stiffness of the MP joint owing to tensioning the FHB.

Once the elevated first ray has been addressed with a correction of its sagittal alignment, the posture and range of motion of the hallux at the first MP joint is evaluated with the ankle in a plantigrade position. If the first MP joint dorsiflexion is

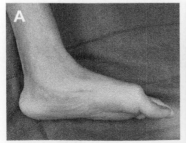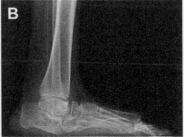

Fig. 5. (*A, B*) Preoperative photo and radiograph of a patient with a symptomatic dorsal bunion. Elevation of the first metatarsal is caused by over pull by the anterior tibial tendon resulting in a contracture of the flexor hallucis brevis. For this patient, motion of the hallux metatarsophalangeal joint was important and therefore a reconstruction was performed without fusion of the metatarsophalangeal joint.

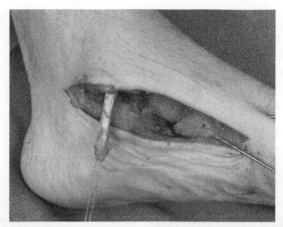

Fig. 6. Reconstruction of the dorsal bunion commences with release of the main deforming force, the anterior tibial tendon. It is transferred laterally once the realignment of the first ray has been completed. The symptomatic dorsal subluxation of the talonavicular joint was addressed with fusion of the talonavicular and medial naviculocuneiform joints with restoration of Meary's angle.

adequate without undue tension of the FHB, transfer of the anterior tibial tendon is performed. When the tension in the FHB is such that dorsiflexion is limited, further shortening or plantar flexion is desired. The authors typically perform a shortening oblique osteotomy of the first metatarsal head. This procedure is an oblique extra-articular osteotomy of the first metatarsal that moves the metatarsal head plantar-ward and proximally. The additional shortening allows for further relaxation of the FHB. If further dorsiflexion is needed, a Moberg osteotomy of the proximal phalanx of the hallux improves the sagittal position of the toe without actually changing the MP joint arc of motion (**Fig. 7**). In cases where there is significant hallux MP joint stiffness, a fusion of the joint gives reliable correction of the deformity. Even with a fusion of the hallux MP joint, it is still necessary to transfer the anterior tibial tendon and address the elevated first metatarsal to achieve adequate alignment and avoid recurrent deformity (**Fig. 8**).

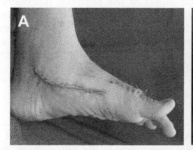
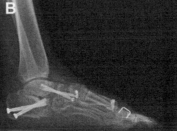

Fig. 7. (A, B) Postoperative photo and radiograph of the same patient as in **Fig. 6**. The postoperative lateral radiograph shows the functional position and arc of motion that was restored to the hallux by plantar flexion and shortening osteotomies of the first meta-tarsal augmented with a Moberg osteotomy of the hallux proximal phalanx. Valgus of the hindfoot was addressed with a medializing calcaneal osteotomy and the arthritic and subluxated talonavicular joint was fused.

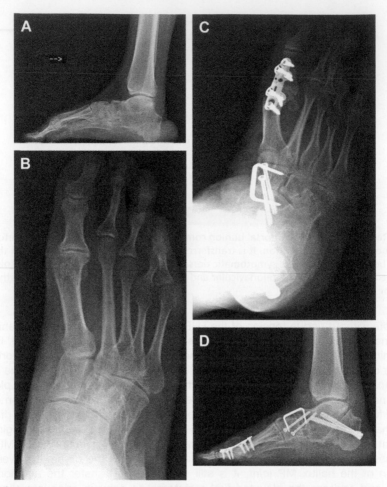

Fig. 8. (*A–D*): Preoperative and postoperative radiographs of a 41-year-old patient with a symptomatic dorsal bunion after prior correction of the clubfoot with a triple arthrodesis. She also complained of chronic pain under the plantar aspect of her heel. Note the elevated first ray and small but very prominent plantar aspect of the posterior tuberosity (*A, B*). Correction was obtained by transfer of the anterior tibial tendon, and plantar flexion of the first ray by removing a plantar wedge and fusion of the medial naviculocuneiform joint. The hindfoot valgus was addressed with a medializing calcaneal osteotomy with an additional closing wedge to reduce the heel prominence (*C*). The dorsal bunion was treated with fusion of the metatarsophalangeal joint (*D*).

Dorsal Subluxation of the Navicular

Subluxation of the navicular is seen exclusively in postoperative clubfeet. It results from an attempt to correct the plantar medial orientation of the navicular on the talar head, which characterizes the cavus deformity seen in clubfeet. The navicular is thicker medially than laterally and, with release of the medial talonavicular ligaments and capsule only, an attempted reduction in a dorsal direction results in rotation around the lateral unreleased talonavicular ligaments. This release causes a rotational deformity of the navicular to a dorsal and medial position on the talar head. Elevation of the thicker medial side of the navicular gives it a wedge-shaped appearance on a lateral radiograph.[18]

This deformity is seen most commonly in the setting of a residual clubfoot with persistent cavus and hindfoot varus. However, in the case of overcorrection, it is associated with hindfoot valgus and arthritic change in the talonavicular joint. A variable amount of subluxation can be found; in severe cases, there is marked plantar flexion of the talar head akin to a congenital vertical talus. On examination, a palpable prominence is present where the navicular is subluxated dorsally. Tenderness of the joint is indicative of degeneration, a common finding that is confirmed on radiographs.

The treatment algorithm here accounts for the severity of the patient's deformity and the presence of symptoms or signs of subtalar arthritis as found with clinical examinations and radiographs. In the absence of subtalar arthritis and with passively correctable valgus, a talonavicular arthrodesis is performed with a medializing calcaneus osteotomy. In more severe and especially rigid deformities with subtalar involvement or signs of subfibular impingement, the authors include the talonavicular joint as part of a triple arthrodesis.

The outcomes of previous attempts at open reduction of the talonavicular joint were not encouraging and are therefore not recommended.[19,20] Multiple authors have found favorable outcomes when a talonavicular arthrodesis is performed for dorsomedial subluxation with persistent deformity after clubfoot surgery.[21,22] Mubarak and colleagues reported on 13 patients (age range, 6–17 years) in whom a talonavicular fusion was performed for symptomatic talonavicular subluxation.[22] All patients had been treated with previous complete posteromedial release. The average follow-up was 3 years with 12 of the 13 patient's symptom free at final follow-up. After surgery, they found a correction of talonavicular subluxation from 42% to 6% using measurement from a lateral weight-bearing radiograph. In addition, they found a restoration of the talo–first metatarsal angle and the calcaneal pitch. They concluded that talonavicular arthrodesis realigns the medial column allowing for normal weight distribution under the forefoot, but that long-term follow-up is needed to assess the effect on the naviculocuneiform joints. An arthrodesis of the talonavicular joint will not correct the elevation of the first metatarsal, which still requires a lateral transfer of the anterior tibial tendon and other maneuvers to correct the elevates, as described.

Flat Top Talus

Flattening of the talar dome is one of the hallmarks of deformity seen in clubfeet (**Fig. 9**). The exact cause has not been defined. Intuitively, one expects that it is caused by the

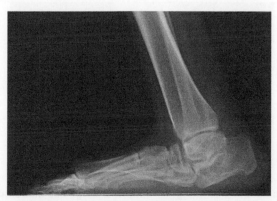

Fig. 9. Weight bearing lateral radiographs of a clubfoot with a flat top talus.

pressure exerted across the tibiotalar joint with forced dorsiflexion during cast treatment, but little evidence exists to support this. A duration of manipulation and casting of longer than 3 months may be contributory.[23,24] An association with peritalar surgical release has also been found, but the exact mechanism is as yet undetermined.[25]

Flattening of the talus is seen as a spectrum of involvement ranging from minimal loss of sphericity to almost complete flattening of the talar dome. Some degree of talar flattening was found in up to 74% of clubfeet, but gross flattening was reported to be present in only 1.5% of cases in 1 series. The degree of flattening seems to strongly influence ankle motion, which in turn is among the major factors influencing functional outcome.[26] The abnormal spherical shape of the talar dome results in abnormal hinge like motion instead of the normal rolling and gliding ankle joint motion (**Fig. 10**). It seems that this deformity is already present at birth and, despite some improvements that may be obtained with Achilles tendon lengthening and soft tissue release, the ultimate outcome of ankle motion may be predetermined by the degree of talar dysplasia present.[27,28] Anterior ankle impingement with prominent osteophytes is a common finding. It has been our experience, however, that anterior cheilectomy does little to improve this deformity, because the osteophytes are indicative of the underlying arthritis and abnormal motion. A cheilectomy does not address this situation, and therefore the symptoms and motion do not improve significantly after cheilectomy; indeed, in these authors' experience, the slight increase in motion increases crepitus and pain and this procedure is rarely indicated.

Treatment of end-stage ankle arthritis in the setting of a clubfoot is challenging. Maintaining motion in the ankle would be ideal and theoretically this could protect more distal joints from added mechanical load and further degeneration. However, when conservative measures fail to address symptomatic ankle arthritis, these authors have found that arthrodesis of the ankle or an ankle replacement to be a very realistic and reliable treatment option, knowing that the patient is at risk of adjacent joint arthritis.

In an attempt to decrease anterior impingement and improve ankle range of motion, Knupp and colleagues[29] performed a supramalleolar tibial osteotomy in 14 adult patients. All had calcaneofibular impingement with hindfoot valgus with additional anterior ankle impingement present in 5 of them. In the cases where combined lateral calcaneofibular and anterior impingement was present a biplanar osteotomy was performed as an anterolateral closing wedge osteotomy. The mean total ankle range of motion for all patients in the study showed a statistically significant improvement

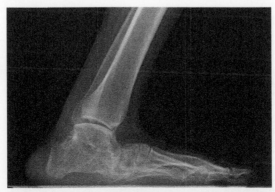

Fig. 10. Lateral radiograph illustrating the abnormal hinge like motion of the ankle joint seen commonly in association with a flat top talus.

from a mean of 25° to 29°. The authors do not agree with the reported outcome of the true range of motion of the ankle in this group of patients. Strictly speaking, it is not possible to obtain any increase in the range of motion because the concept of improving motion by performing an osteotomy is that seen in a Moberg osteotomy of the hallux proximal phalanx. Rather than improving the total arc of motion, it serves to bring the existing range of motion into a different plane. Although this may be useful to obtain a plantigrade foot in the presence of an equinus deformity of the ankle, it cannot improve actual motion in an abnormal joint.

A total ankle replacement in the setting of a clubfoot is an interesting concept, but there are several salient points that complicate this procedure. To begin with, the abnormal hinged ankle motion that gave rise to the joint degeneration is likely to persist owing to the abnormal posterior soft tissue envelope. This includes the Achilles tendon, posterior tibial tendon, and posterior capsule that may be severely scarred secondary to multiple surgeries and will limit the potential range of motion that could be obtained. In addition to that, several anatomic factors need to be taken into account such as the small and narrow talus, the posterior position of the fibula, and thus the small surface area for the prosthesis. Nonetheless, this treatment remains a viable alternative for managing these deformities, particularly when some ankle range of motion is desirable. Keep in mind, however, that this procedure can only be performed in the presence of a plantigrade foot, so that the replacement should be staged after correction of the forefoot and hindfoot deformity.

SUMMARY

The overcorrected clubfoot is a complication seen after surgical release of the foot. Despite the infrequency with which the posteromedial release is performed today, this entity presents occasionally to the orthopedic foot and ankle surgeon. A sound understanding of the underlying muscle imbalance is essential when addressing the resulting deformities. The surgical aim is to provide the patient with a pain-free, stable, and plantigrade foot that is in neutral alignment. Preserving joint motion is preferable, but not always possible. Several distinct deformities are seen commonly and our treatment algorithm for these was discussed. The underlying pathoanatomy, which includes the skeletal and soft tissue structures, complicates treatment and necessitates a different approach. As the body of literature dealing with the overcorrected clubfoot continues to expand, it will aid the treating surgeon to achieve an optimal outcome with great benefit to the patient.

REFERENCES

1. van Gelder JH, van Ruiten AG, Visser JD, et al. Long-term results of the posteromedial release in the treatment of idiopathic clubfoot. J Pediatr Orthop 2010; 30(7):700–4.
2. Ponseti IV, Campos J. Observations on pathogenesis and treatment of congenital clubfoot. Clin Orthop Relat Res 1972;84:50–60.
3. Laaveg SJ, Ponseti IV. Long-term results of treatment of congenital club foot. J Bone Joint Surg Am 1980;62(1):23–31.
4. Cooper DM, Dietz FR. Treatment of idiopathic clubfoot. A thirty-year follow-up note. J Bone Joint Surg Am 1995;77(10):1477–89.
5. Ippolito E, Farsetti P, Caterini R, et al. Long-term comparative results in patients with congenital clubfoot treated with two different protocols. J Bone Joint Surg Am 2003;85-A(7):1286–94.

6. Morcuende JA, Dolan LA, Dietz FR, et al. Radical reduction in the rate of extensive corrective surgery for clubfoot using the Ponseti method. Pediatrics 2004; 113(2):376–80.

7. Boehm S, Limpaphayom N, Alaee F, et al. Early results of the Ponseti method for the treatment of clubfoot in distal arthrogryposis. J Bone Joint Surg Am 2008; 90(7):1501–7.

8. Gurnett CA, Boehm S, Connolly A, et al. Impact of congenital talipes equinovarus etiology on treatment outcomes. Dev Med Child Neurol 2008;50(7): 498–502.

9. Feldbrin Z, Gilai AN, Ezra E, et al. Muscle imbalance in the aetiology of idiopathic club foot. An electromyographic study. J Bone Joint Surg Br 1995;77(4): 596–601.

10. Stevens PM, Otis S. Ankle valgus and clubfeet. J Pediatr Orthop 1999;19(4): 515–7.

11. Turco VJ. Resistant congenital club foot—one-stage posteromedial release with internal fixation. A follow-up report of a fifteen-year experience. J Bone Joint Surg Am 1979;61(6):805–14.

12. Simons GW. The complete subtalar release in clubfeet [review]. Orthop Clin North Am 1987;18(4):667–88.

13. Cohen-Sobel E, Caselli M, Giorgini R, et al. Long-term follow-up of clubfoot surgery: analysis of 44 patients [review]. J Foot Ankle Surg 1993;32(4):411–23.

14. Hudson I, Catterall A. Posterolateral release for resistant club foot. J Bone Joint Surg Br 1994;76(2):281–4.

15. Ponseti IV. Congenital clubfoot: fundamentals of treatment. Oxford (United Kingdom): Oxford University Press; 1996.

16. Thompson GH, Hoyen HA, Barthel T. Tibialis anterior tendon transfer after clubfoot surgery. Clin Orthop Relat Res 2009;467(5):1306–13.

17. McKay DW. Dorsal bunions in children. J Bone Joint Surg Am 1983;65(7):975–80.

18. Kuo KN, Jansen LD. Rotatory dorsal subluxation of the navicular: a complication of clubfoot surgery. J Pediatr Orthop 1998;18(6):770–4.

19. Barnett RM Sr. Medial/lateral column separation (third street operation) for dorsal talonavicular subluxation. In: Simons GW, editor. The clubfoot: the present and view of the future. New York: Springer-Verlag; 1994. p. 268–72.

20. Schlafly B, Butler JE, Siff SJ, et al. The appearance of the tarsal navicular after posteromedial release for clubfoot. Foot Ankle 1985;5(5):222–37.

21. Wei SY, Sullivan RJ, Davidson RS. Talo-navicular arthrodesis for residual midfoot deformities of a previously corrected clubfoot. Foot Ankle Int 2000;21(6): 482–5.

22. Swaroop VT, Wenger DR, Mubarak SJ. Talonavicular fusion for dorsal subluxation of the navicular in resistant clubfoot. Clin Orthop Relat Res 2009;467(5): 1314–8.

23. Sullivan RJ, Davidson RS. When does the flat-top talus lesion occur in idiopathic clubfoot: evaluation with magnetic resonance imaging at three months of age. Foot Ankle Int 2001;22(5):422–5.

24. Mahmoodian R, Leasure J, Gadikota H, et al. Mechanical properties of human fetal talus. Clin Orthop Relat Res 2009;467:1186–94.

25. Pinto JA, Hernandes AC, Buchaim TP, et al. Radiographic abnormalities of the talus in patients with clubfoot after surgical release using the McKay technique. Rev Bras Ortop 2011;46(3):293–8. ISSN 0102-3616.

26. Hutchins PM, Foster BK, Paterson DC, et al. Long-term results of early surgical release in club feet. J Bone Joint Surg Br 1985;67(5):791–9.

27. Hjelmstedt EA, Sahlstedt B. Arthrography as a guide in the treatment of congenital clubfoot. Findings and treatment results in a consecutive series. Acta Orthop Scand 1980;51(2):321–34.
28. Dunn HK, Samuelson KM. Flat-top talus. A long-term report of twenty club feet. J Bone Joint Surg Am 1975;56(1):57–62.
29. Knupp M, Barg A, Bolliger L, et al. Reconstructive surgery for overcorrected clubfoot in adults. J Bone Joint Surg Am 2012;94(15):e1101.

Tendon Transfers Around the Foot: When and Where

Ken N. Kuo, MD[a,b,c,]*, Kuan-Wen Wu, MD[b],
Joseph J. Krzak, PhD, PT, PCS[d,e], Peter A. Smith, MD[c,e]

KEYWORDS

- Anterior tibial tendon transfer • Posterior tibial tendon transfer
- Reverse Jones transfer • Peabody transfer

KEY POINTS

- Fixed and dynamic foot deformities in children are often caused by tendon imbalance of 4 motion components of the foot and ankle: dorsiflexion, plantar flexion, eversion, and inversion.
- Passively correctable ankle and foot range of motion is essential before tendon transfer as the transfer only holds the corrected deformity and improves balance and function.
- Anterior tibial tendon transfer, either full or split, is commonly used in children with clubfoot and cerebral palsy to correct forefoot supination in the swing phase.
- Posterior tibial tendon transfer to the dorsum of the foot is helpful in drop foot deformity of different causes, such as Charcot-Marie-Tooth disease or peroneal nerve palsy.
- Reverse jones transfer is useful to correct the dorsal bunion deformity.
- Peabody transfer is employed in patients with calcaneus type of gait.

INTRODUCTION

Children's foot deformities are often caused by imbalance of neuromuscular function. The most common deformities are varus, valgus, equinus, and calcaneus. Correspondingly, there are 4 essential motions that dominate the function of the ankle, plantar flexion, dorsiflexion, inversion, and eversion. Motor imbalance not only causes functional disability but it can also cause a fixed foot deformity with growth. Therefore, once a particular pattern of imbalance is established, tendon transfers are common procedures

The authors have nothing to disclose.
[a] Center for Evidence-Based Medicine, Taipei Medical University, 250 Wuxing Street, Taipei 11031, Taiwan; [b] Department of Orthopaedic Surgery, National Taiwan University Hospital, 7 Chung Shan South Road, Taipei 10002, Taiwan; [c] Department of Orthopaedic Surgery, Rush University Medical Center, 1725 West Harrison, Chicago, IL 60612, USA; [d] Physical Therapy Program, College of Health Sciences, Midwestern University, 555 31st Street, Downers Grove, IL 60515, USA; [e] Shriners Hospital for Children, 2211 North Oak Park Avenue, Chicago, IL 60707, USA
* Corresponding author. 250 Wuxing Street, Taipei 11031, Taiwan.
E-mail address: kennank@aol.com

in the treatment of pediatric foot and ankle deformities. Tendon transfer around the foot in children serves the primary purpose of balancing the function or in some instances serves as a tether of the motion in a more functional position if desirable active function does not occur. In almost any musculotendinous unit, a combination can be selected for transfer; but there are a few common transfers that satisfy the requirements for a successful result. Several procedures have been reported for different deformities.

There are several essential points in tendon transfer.

- First, there must be adequate motor power for the transferred tendon. As a rule of thumb, reverse phase tendon transfers usually lose one grade of motor function by the Jones classification (examination for muscle strength commonly used in pediatric orthopedic field, consists of 5 grades); this is not the case for tendon transfers in the same phasic pattern.
- Second, the foot should be at the neutral and plantar grade position. Tendon transfers do not correct the deformity; they can only hold the corrected deformity. If there is an existing deformity, it should be corrected before surgery, either through soft tissue or bony procedures.
- Third, a good passive range of motion is desirable for better results.
- Fourth, there must be adequate length of the donor tendon to be transferred to provide an effective functional length and allow adequate extension.

The procedures usually require multiple skin incisions that enable tendon passage under intact skin.

Often, the tendon transferred is anchored to the bone to house the end of the donor tendon. There are 2 common ways to fix the tendon in bone.

- The end of the donor tendon is tagged with a suture. The suture is passed through a hole in the bone and comes out the bottom of the foot. By pulling both ends of the suture in desirable tension, the sutures are tightened on a sterile button at the plantar surface of the foot or tied against the plantar fascia.
- Instead of using a button, there are recent reports of using bioabsorbable screws to anchor the tendon at the bone hole.[1] This method can only be used for larger children.

SURGICAL TECHNIQUE
Anterior Tibial Tendon Transfer

Anterior tibial tendon transfer (ATTT) is the earliest described procedure. In 1940, Garceau[2] first described ATTT and reported excellent results. In Ponseti's[3] earlier publication of their eponymous method, the ATTT was a rather popular procedure. In 1974, Hoffer and colleagues[4] described split anterior tibia ten transfer (SPLATT) in children with cerebral palsy. The split transfer procedure has also been expanded for the management of residual clubfoot deformity.[5] It is a simple procedure with a predictable outcome.

Indications

- Residual flexible clubfoot with intoeing, dynamic supination, and forefoot adduction during gait (best age for the procedure is around 4 to 6 years old).
- In combination with soft tissue release in recurrent or untreated clubfoot deformity
- Diplegic cerebral palsy with equinus foot and forefoot adduction, usually in combination with gastrocnemius lengthening
- Absent peroneal muscle function from other diseases, such as trauma or neuropathy with some remaining AT tendon function causing an imbalance

Preoperative planning
The patients' foot should achieve a passive range of motion to neutral position. Patients demonstrate AT tendon function, which is out of balance with the other dorsiflexion evident by gait observation. Specifically, the forefoot assures a supination position during the swing phase with impaired clearance or lands on the lateral aspect of the foot. It is desirable that muscle strength of the AT tendon is at least 4. This strength can be evaluated by asking the child to walk on their heels.

Prep and patient positioning
Patients are placed in a supine position. A tourniquet is applied.

Surgical approach and procedure
Full ATTT:

- The first incision is at the medial dorsal aspect at the junction of medial cuneiform bone and first metatarsal.
- Expose the AT tendon and transect at the insertion, and tag the end of the tendon with a polyglactin 910 (Vicryl) suture (**Fig. 1**A).
- The second incision is at the anterior aspect of the lower leg at the lateral border of the tibia about 4 to 5 cm above the ankle joint line. Incise the tendon sheath to expose the AT tendon, and then deliver the transected tendon to the proximal wound (**Fig. 1**B). A tendon passer or Luque wire is useful to pass the suture in order to keep the tendon within the proper compartment.
- The third incision is at the middle or third cuneiform on the dorsum of the foot. The end of the tendon is passed subcutaneously to the third incision using a large hemostat (**Fig. 1**C).
- After the lateral cuneiform is exposed, a drill hole is made through the bone (**Fig. 1**D).
- Using a straight needle, the suture ends are passed through the hole and exit through a felt pad and button at the bottom of the foot. It is then tightened to the button in maximum tension with the foot in dorsiflexion (**Fig. 1**E). Usually the suture is tied after closure of all skin incisions.

Split anterior tibial tendon transfer
- At the first incision, expose the AT tendon at its insertion, where the distal end of the tendon is often naturally split. The lateral half is isolated with a looped No. 1 nylon suture, which is passed to the proximal incision and used to complete the split. The half tendon (lateral half) attached to the medial cuneiform is transected. The end is tagged with a Vicryl stitch using a Bunnell technique (**Fig. 2**A).
- The half tendon is pulled proximally at the second incision, either by pulling on the nylon suture or passing the Bunnell suture up to the proximal incision after passing with a tendon passer or a Luque wire. The tendon will split evenly as it is pulled proximally (**Fig. 2**B).
- The third incision is on top of the cuboid or cuneiform depending on where balance is achieved. The end of tendon is passed subcutaneously to the third incision using a large hemostat (**Fig. 2**C).
- A drill hole is made through the cuboid or cuneiform (**Fig. 2**D).
- Using a straight needle, the sutures are passed through the hole to the bottom of the foot and tightened over a felt pad and button in maximum tension with the foot in dorsiflexion (see **Fig. 1**E).

604

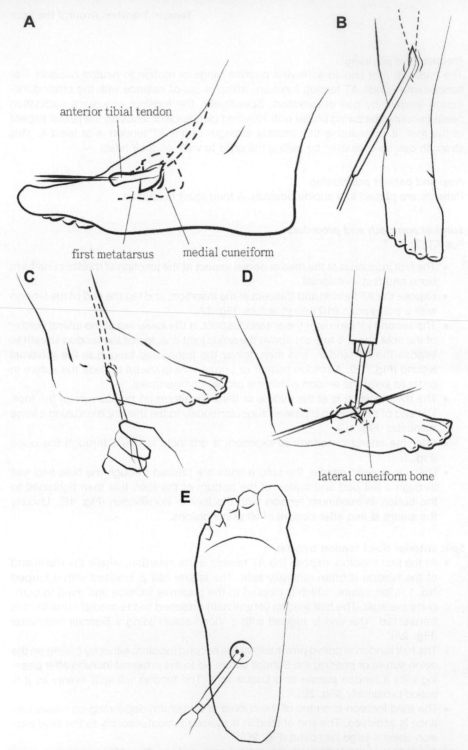

anterior tibial tendon

first metatarsus   medial cuneiform

lateral cuneiform bone

Fig. 1. Full ATTT. (*A*) Expose the AT tendon and transect at the insertion; tag the end of the tendon with a Vicryl suture. (*B*) Deliver the transected tendon to the proximal wound. (*C*) The end of the tendon is passed subcutaneously to the third incision using a large hemostat. (*D*) A drill hole is made through the bone. (*E*) The sutures are tightened to the button in maximum tension with the foot in dorsiflexion.

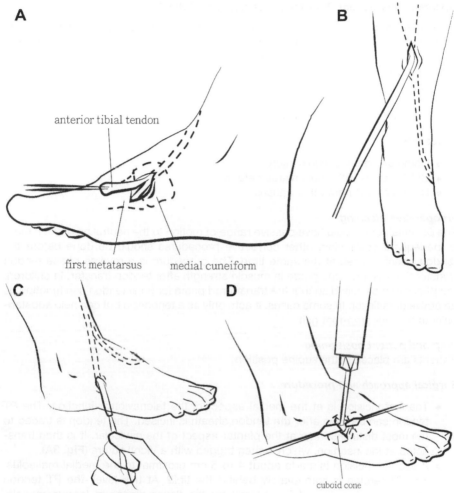

A

anterior tibial tendon

first metatarsus   medial cuneiform

B

C

D

cuboid cone

Fig. 2. SPLATT. (*A*) The lateral half of the tendon attached to the medial cuneiform is transected. (*B*) The tendon will split evenly as it is pulled proximally. (*C*) The end of the tendon is passed subcutaneously to the third incision. (*D*) A drill hole is made through the cuboid or cuneiform.

Immediate postoperative care

- A short walking leg cast is applied for 6 weeks with the foot in neutral position with applied dorsiflexion and eversion.

Rehabilitation and recovery

- After cast removal, use a hinged ankle-foot orthosis (AFO) with plantar flexion stopped at 90° and free dorsiflexion for 6 months, during gait.

Possible pitfalls of ATTT are as follows:

- The tendon is not tensioned when it is tightened to the drill hole with the foot in dorsiflexion.
- There is possibility that ATTT may overcorrect varus into valgus with time in long-term follow-up of quadriplegic or diplegic spastic cerebral palsy children.

Posterior Tibial Tendon Transfer to the Dorsum of the Foot

When there is absence of AT and/or peroneal tendon function, drop-foot gait is usually the symptom that causes walking difficulty. It often occurs in common peroneal nerve damage or loss of anterior compartment muscle caused by compartment syndrome. It can be a presentation of a progressive neuromuscular disease like Charcot-Marie-Tooth (CMT) disease or muscular dystrophy. The posterior tibial (PT) tendon becomes a deforming factor. The loss of function causes imbalanced muscle strength around the ankle with progressive equinovarus deformity.

Indications

- Common peroneal nerve injury
- CMT disease with equinovarus deformity
- Drop-foot gait from other causes

Preoperative planning

The patients' foot should have passive range of motion to the neutral position. If there is inadequate positioning, other corrective procedures should be done before the tendon transfer, often at the same time. The procedure is a reverse phase tendon transfer that can lose one grade in muscle strength after tendon transfer. In children, the phase can be suited so that the transferred posterior tibial tendon can function as an active dorsiflexor. In some cases, it acts only as a tenodesis but can help substantially to prevent drop-foot gait.

Prep and patient positioning

Patients are placed in the supine position.

Surgical approach and procedure

- The first incision is at the medial aspect of the talonavicular junction. The PT tendon can be seen after the tendon sheath is incised. The tendon is traced to the most distal insertion at the plantar aspect of the navicular. It is then transected at the insertion, which is then tagged with a Vicryl suture (**Fig. 3**A).
- A second incision is made about 4 to 5 cm proximal to the medial malleolus. The PT tendon is immediately behind the tibia. At this level, the PT tendon often goes deeper and is covered by the flexor digitorum longus muscle. The tendon is then pulled through proximally (**Fig. 3**B). It may be necessary to trim the stump of the detached tendon or release the sheath of the ankle to allow passage.
- A third incision is made along the anterior aspect of the tibia on the lateral edge about 5 to 6 cm proximal to the ankle joint line. Using a large curved hemostat along the tibia above the periosteum, an instrument is passed from the lateral side of the tibia, penetrating the interosseous membrane, and then curving around posterior aspect of tibia until entering the posterior medial aspect of the tibia at the second incision (**Fig. 3**C). The tendon is pulled into the third incision. Caution is taken not to include soft tissue while penetrating with the hemostat, so no damage is made to the muscular and neurovascular structures.
- A fourth incision is made at the middle or lateral cuneiform bones on the dorsum of the foot depending on the degree of varus deformity. The tendon is then passed subcutaneously using a large hemostat (**Fig. 3**D). It is important to widen the subcutaneous tunnel using a hemostat for the passage of the tendon.
- An adequate drill hole is made at the cuneiform (**Fig. 3**E).

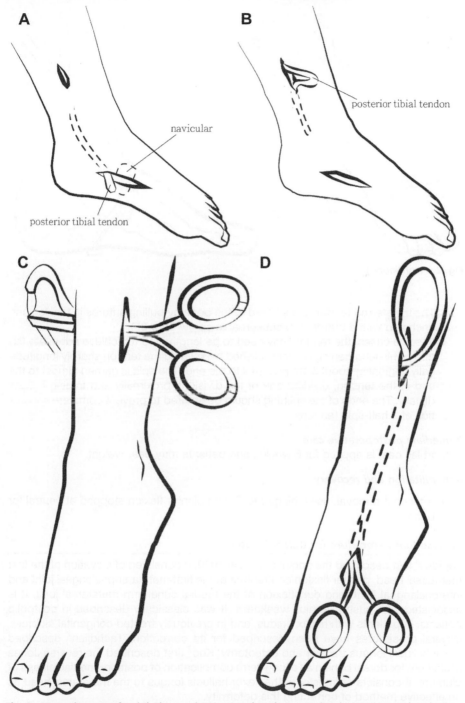

Fig. 3. PT tendon transfer. (*A*) The tendon is traced to the most distal insertion at the plantar aspect of the navicular and transected at insertion. (*B*) The tendon is pulled through proximally. (*C*) Using a large curved hemostat to penetrate the interosseous membrane from the anterior lateral to posterior medial aspect to bring the tendon anteriorly. (*D*) The tendon is then passed subcutaneously distally. (*E*) A drill hole is made at the cuneiform. (*F*) The transferred tendon is anchored to the bone.

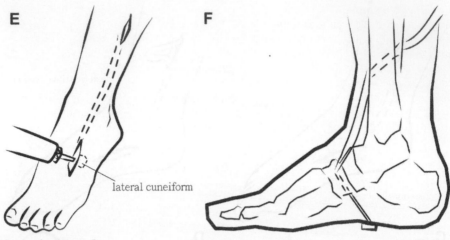

lateral cuneiform

Fig. 3. (*continued*)

- The transferred tendon is anchored to the bone by pulling sutures in tension and anchored with a button or bioabsorbable screw (**Fig. 3**F).
- In some cases, the tendon may need to be lengthened to achieve adequate fixation. This lengthening is accomplished by splitting the tendon sharply longitudinally beginning about 5 cm proximal to the end. The split is carried almost to the end of the tendon, dividing one of the divisions proximally and folding it back distally. The ends of the splitting should be sutured to prevent complete separation of 2 half-split tendons.

Immediate postoperative care
A short leg cast is applied for 6 weeks, and patients may bear weight.

Rehabilitation and recovery

- After cast removal, use a hinged AFO with plantar flexion stopped at neutral for 6 months.

Reverse Jones Procedure for Dorsal Bunion

Lapidus[6] first described the dorsal bunion in 1940. It consisted of elevation of the first metatarsal head, plantar flexion contracture at the first metatarsophalangeal joint and interphalangeal joint, and dorsiflexion of the medial cuneiform-metatarsal joint. It is associated with gastrocnemius weakness. It was classically described in postpolio patients, in patients with hallux rigidus, and in previously treated congenital clubfeet. Several procedures have been described for its correction. Tachdjian[7] described flexor hallucis longus transfer and osteotomy. Kuo[7] first described the reverse Jones procedure for dorsal bunion as a long-term complication of posterior medial release of clubfoot. It consists of transfer of the flexor hallucis longus to the metatarsal head as an effective method of correcting this deformity.

Indications

- After posterior medial release for clubfoot, when deformity develops with difficulty in shoe wear and pain
- Postpolio cases

Preoperative planning
The great toe of the foot is in hyperflexion at the metatarsophalangeal joint. The first metatarsal head is in a dorsiflexion position that forms a dorsal prominence. The function of the flexor hallucis longus should be active and graded 4 or 5. The ankle joint can be passively placed in the neutral position. Often the dorsal bunion cannot be reduced to an anatomic position passively. For the best result in this situation, a simultaneous proximal first metatarsal plantar flexion osteotomy should be performed in the same setting. In those with forefoot supination during the gait and overpuling of the AT tendon, a simultaneous ATTT should be performed.

Prep and patient positioning
Patients are placed in the supine position. A tourniquet is applied for facilitating the surgery.

Surgical approach and procedure

- The incision is carried out along the medial aspect of the great toe from the interphalangeal joint, extending proximally about 1 cm proximal to the neck of the metatarsal (**Fig. 4**A).
- Through the incision, go to the plantar aspect, and the flexor hallucis longus is explored. It is traced to the insertion at the proximal end of the distal phalanx.
- The flexor hallucis longus is then transected; leave a 1.5-cm stump for tenodesis to the flexor hallucis brevis by suturing side to side (**Fig. 4**B).
- The free end of the flexor hallucis longus is tagged with Vicryl using a Bunnell tendon suture technique. Then the end of tendon is free up to the proximal end of the incision. The tendon is passed under the soft tissue to the medial side of first metatarsal against the bone (**Fig. 4**C).
- A drill bit of adequate size for the donor tendon is used to drill vertically at the junction of the metatarsal head and neck (**Fig. 4**D).
- Using a long needle, the free ends of the sutures are pulled through the hole from the plantar surface to the dorsal side of the metatarsal bone (**Fig. 4**E).
- If necessary, a closed wedge plantar flexion osteotomy of the proximal first metatarsal is performed and fixed with a staple or Kirschner wires.
- Placing the foot in plantar flexion for maximum tension, the end of the tendon is sutured back to itself (**Fig. 4**F). Check the tension of the transfer.

Immediate postoperative care

- A short walking leg cast is applied for 6 weeks.

Rehabilitation and recovery

- After cast removal, there is no special need for rehabilitation.

Peabody Procedure in Myelomeningocele

In patients with myelomeningocele, there are many variations of foot deformity depending on the level of involvement. Calcaneal foot deformity typically occurs in L4 level involvement with the AT tendon the sole functioning muscle in the foot. The deformity is progressive. It causes heel ulcerations because the heel is the only weight-bearing point. Posterior transfer of the AT tendon to the calcaneus is a good way to correct and prevent the deformity. It may not produce a functional push off; however, by taking away the deforming factor and tethering the plantar flexion, function is sufficient to produce a good result. There is evidence that younger patients have a better functional result from this procedure, but it can be performed at any age in childhood.

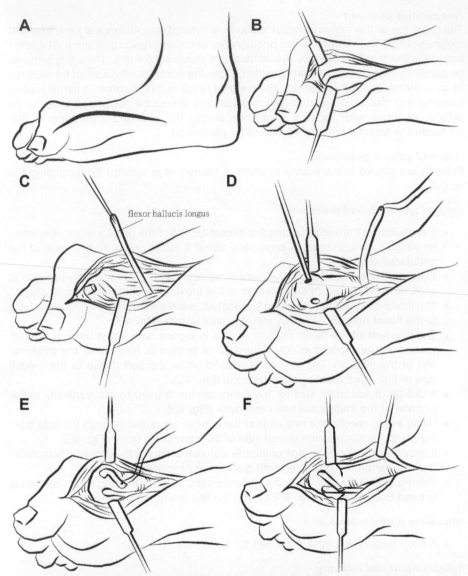

Fig. 4. Reverse Jones transfer. (*A*) The incision is on the medial aspect of the great toe proximally to about 1 cm proximal to the neck of the metatarsal. (*B*) The flexor hallucis longus is then transected. (*C*) The tendon is passed under the soft tissue to the medial side of the first metatarsal. (*D*) A drill hall is made vertically at the junction of the metatarsal head and neck. (*E*) Using a long straight needle, the free ends of the sutures are pulled through the hole from plantar to dorsal and carry the tendon through the drill hole. (*F*) The end of the tendon is sutured back to itself with tension while placing the foot in the plantar flexion position.

Indications

- Calcaneal foot deformity in patients with myelomeningocele with the AT tendon being the only functioning muscle

Preoperative planning
The foot is in the calcaneal position. The AT tendon serves as the only functioning muscle or tethering tendon. Also, the ankle joint may be passively manipulated to the neutral position.

Prep and patient positioning
Patients are placed in the supine position. It is necessary to apply a tourniquet for facilitating the surgery.

Surgical approach and procedure

- The first incision is at the insertion of the AT tendon at the navicular first metatarsal junction on the medial dorsal aspect. The tendon sheath is opened and the tendon is isolated. Make sure there is no other soft tissue attached. The tendon is transected at the insertion, and the end is tagged with a Vicryl suture using the Bunnell technique (**Fig. 5A**).
- The second incision is at the anterior tibia aspect about 4 to 5 cm proximal to the ankle joint. The AT tendon sheath is opened, and the tendon is identified. The distal end of the tendon is then pulled to the proximal wound (**Fig. 5B**).
- The third incision is carried out at the posterior aspect of the ankle medial to the Achilles tendon all the way down to the calcaneal bone (**Fig. 5C**). Soft tissue at the medial side of Achilles tendon is dissected all the way down to the posterior aspect of the tibia bone.
- From the anterior tibia aspect, using a large hemostat, a tract is made from anterior to posterior against the lateral bone surface of the tibia. Once the tip of the hemostat appears at the posterior wound, the tract is made large enough for the tendon to pass through by repeat opening of the hemostat. Then, use another hemostat to trace the track from the back. Once it goes through, grab the end of tagged suture and pull the tendon posteriorly (**Fig. 5D**).
- A drill hole is made in the posterior aspect of the calcaneal bone next to the Achilles tendon insertion. Using a straight needle, the tag suture is pulled to the bottom of the foot. The tendon is then pulled into the hole and tightened on a button (**Fig. 5E**). Optionally, the transferred tendon may be sutured to the Achilles tendon side to side.

Immediate postoperative care

- A short leg walking cast is applied for 6 weeks.

Rehabilitation and recovery

- After cast removal, a solid AFO is applied.
- Rehabilitate for training of the muscle function in the new location.

CLINICAL RESULTS IN THE LITERATURES
Anterior Tibial Tendon Transfer

Overactivity of the AT muscle or a normal AT function with weak antagonist, particularly the peroneal muscles, may cause a varus foot deformity. This sequela is common following treatment of congenital talipes equinovarus deformities, vascular hemiplegia, or other neurologic disorders. This abnormal position of the foot causes alterations of the

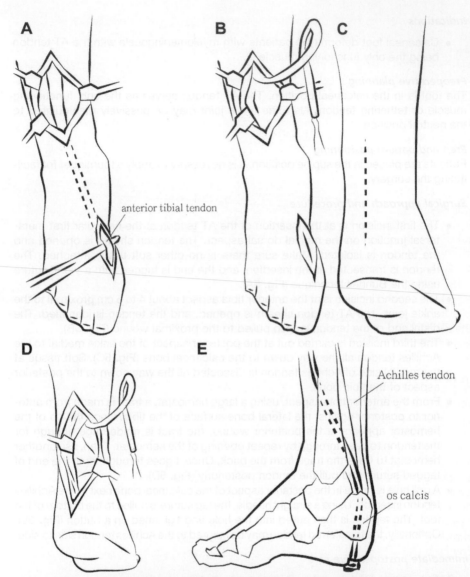

Fig. 5. Peabody transfer. (*A*) The AT tendon is transected at the insertion. (*B*) The detached tendon is then pulled to the proximal wound. (*C*) The third incision is carried out at the posterior aspect of the ankle medial to the Achilles tendon down to the calcaneal bone. (*D*) The AT tendon is passed posteriorly. (*E*) The tendon is pulled into the hole and tightens on a button.

biomechanics of the foot during the gait cycle and can induce a painful callosity on the lateral border of the foot from abnormal weight bearing and also result in poor foot clearance during the swing phase. When physical therapy and bracing fail to maintain a plantigrade position, surgical correction with AT tendon full or split transfer is indicated.

Full Anterior Tibia Tendon Transfer

Residual dynamic forefoot adduction and supination deformities are commonly observed during the course of treatment of congenital clubfoot. The major presenting functional problems are intoeing, tripping, and difficulty in shoe wear. Relatively stronger AT tendon pulling has been recognized as a contributing factor, especially along with weak peroneal muscles. Garceau[2] first described the use of ATTT in recurrent clubfoot deformity. Their series reported 77% good and excellent results in forefoot adduction correction and 93% in inversion deformity correction. Since then, the ATTT has been widely use to manage the recurrent dynamic supination deformity following clubfoot surgery. Kuo and colleagues[5] reported a series of 71 feet in 55 patients, which included 42 full AT transfer and 29 split AT transfer. The average range of surgery was between 4 and 8 years. After detaching from its insertion, the AT tendon was passed subcutaneously and then transplanted to the middle or lateral cuneiform in full transfer, while into the cuboid in a split transfer. Both groups showed clinical improvement according to the Garceau criteria. In the full transfer group, there were 13 excellent, 28 good, and one fair compared with 11 excellent and 18 good in the split transfer group. There was a significant increase of range of motion in dorsiflexion and eversion after tendon transfer. The average gain in eversion strength for both groups was 1.5 grades with significant difference. They concluded that AT transfer is an effective method of correcting a dynamic clubfoot deformity, either with a full or split transfer.

In 2009, Thompson and colleagues[8] described the subcutaneous ATTT for clubfoot deformities and maintained its normal position beneath the ankle retinaculum. This method has the advantage of preserving normal tendon mechanics and prevents the tendon from bowstringing while the foot is in dorsiflexion. Comparable with the results of other studies, they also obtained a high rate of satisfactory results (87%) after ATTT for correcting recurrent clubfoot deformities.

Split Anterior Tibia Tendon Transfer

Spastic equinovarus (SEV) foot is the most common lower limb deformity following traumatic brain injury and cerebral palsy. It is caused by increased tone of the plantar flexor and inversion muscles, which can be the AT muscle, the PT, or the gastrocnemius itself. Lengthening of the Achilles tendon alone, which is used for the equinus foot, does not always correct the varus deformity. To address the problem of muscle imbalance in the equinovarus foot, Hoffer and colleagues,[4] in 1974, originated the surgical procedure of SPLATT for supination and varus deformity of the midfoot in children with cerebral palsy. According to their 10-year follow-up series of SPLATT in 1985, all patients with cerebral palsy with preoperative equinovarus feet showed improved ambulation and discarded the use of orthoses.[9] The reported clinical outcomes of SPLATT have been generally promising. A preliminary result from Wu and colleagues'[1] series in 2009 described 10 excellent and 6 good results without any poor cases by using a bioabsorbable interference screw as a modified fixation technique. The bioabsorbable screws have been shown to have more secure tendon fixation and to prevent potential complications of failure of fixation and rupture of the transferred tendon.

The selection of the appropriate tendon for lengthening or transfer in patients with equinovarus foot is complicated and can be improved with electromyography or foot and ankle motion analysis.[10] The SPLATT may be done in conjunction with a lengthening of the PT and the gastrocnemius for hemiplegic patients with generally good results.[11] However, the use of SPLATT in patients with diplegic and quadriplegic cerebral palsy is cautioned as it may often result in long-term overcorrection of the foot into a valgus or abducted position.[12]

SEV foot deformity accompanied with clawing toes is also the common motor sequel following stroke and traumatic brain injury.[13,14] Brace wear is difficult as dynamic forces of spastic muscles and static soft tissue contractures develop over time. A large series of 177 patients who sustained hemiplegic stroke obtained a significant improvement in foot position, gait function, and forward propulsion with SPLATT.[15] Another study by Hosalkar and colleagues[16] reported that all 47 SEV feet were corrected to plantigrade position and improved the ambulatory status, with 77% of patients discontinuing bracing. The investigators also recommended their modified fixation techniques, changing the original dorsoplantar routing of the cuboid tunnel to lateromedial routing. One important issue before determining SPLATT surgery in adults with neurologic disorders is the appropriate timing of surgery. Recovery of motor function after an upper motor neuron insult can continue for up to 6 to 9 months. Therefore, it is recommended to postpone surgery until after this period.[17]

Posterior Tibial Tendon Transfer to the Dorsum of the Foot

The PT tendon can be transferred through the interosseous membrane anteriorly to the foot dorsum to correct drop-foot deformity caused by irreversible traumatic peroneal nerve palsy, a deficit of dorsiflexor muscles,[18,19] CMT disease,[20] leprosy,[21] and Duchenne muscular dystrophy.[22] After the PT tendon is transferred to the anterior ankle, dorsiflexion is restored and the medial deforming force of the foot is also eliminated. In reviewing the literature, Mayer[23] was the first to use PT tendon transfer in treating patients with posttraumatic peroneal nerve paralysis. Afterward, Watkins and colleagues[24] further described their technique of PT tendon transfer anteriorly through the interosseous membrane to restore the dorsiflexion function of the foot and obtained 24 good or excellent results in 25 patients. Lipscomb and Sanchez[25] also reported good results in 9 of 10 patients who had combined PT tendon transfer and triple arthrodesis for common peroneal nerve palsy. The crucial points of transferring PT tendon include harvesting maximal tendon length, using a subcutaneous course to prevent tendon adhesion, and securing tendon-to-bone fixation. For cases with concomitant AT dysfunction and peroneal tendon weakness, PT tendon transfer to a lateral cuneiform is recommended to antagonize the unopposed inversion force produced from the medial toe flexors.

Several technique modifications have been raised to refine the procedures and assure satisfactory results. In 1968, Srinivasan and colleagues[26] split the PT tendon into 2 tails, with the medial tail inserted into the tendon of extensor hallucis longus and the lateral tail into the tendons of extensor digitorum longus and peroneus tertius. In 1978, Hsu and Hoffer[27] developed a 4-incision technique for PT tendon transfer to minimize the soft tissue dissection. This modified procedure were carried out in 22 patients and had promising results without any complications. For patients with a higher level of neurologic condition, the greater foot deformity is often caused by involving both the anterior and lateral compartments. In 1991, McCall and colleagues[28] proposed the Bridle procedure, a tritendon double-end-weave anastomosis between the PT, AT, and peroneal longus tendon; it may be the best option for flexible equines and equinovarus deformities.

Because a drop-foot deformity is frequently accompanied with equinus contracture, conjunct tendo Achilles lengthening or gastrocnemius recession might be necessarily executed to improve the range of passive dorsiflexion.

CMT disease is recognized as one the most common neurogenic causes of cavovarus deformity and drop foot. This abnormal gait may be affected by weak AT muscle, and the long toe extensors are often concomitantly involved. There are no active dorsiflexors to prevent drop foot in the swing phase of the gait. In this situation, the PT tendon, originally phasic as a plantar-flexor, can act as an active dorsiflexor after being anteriorly transferred to the dorsum of the foot in patients with CMT disease. Dreher and colleagues[20] investigated their series of 23 feet in 14 patients by clinical examination and 3-dimensional gait analysis following PT tendon transfer to correct the drop-foot component. Significant increase in tibiotalar dorsiflexion during the swing phase was shown, accompanied by a decrease in maximum plantar flexion at the stance-swing transition. The American Orthopedic Foot and Ankle Society score also improved significantly. They concluded PT tendon transfer was effective at correcting the foot-drop component of cavovarus foot deformity in patients with CMT.

Drop foot caused by paralysis of the AT and peroneal muscles is found as a common sequel secondary to leprosy. Up to 30% of patients have fixed nerve palsy by the time of diagnosis of leprosy.[29] The possibility of using tendon transfer in leprosy was inspired by the report of Watkins and colleagues[24] who had used PT tendon in poliomyelitis through the interosseous route. Later, several studies reported excellent results after PT tendon transfer through the interosseous route along with elongation of tendo Achilles in treating leprosy-related drop foot. Around 80% of patients were able to produce active dorsiflexion, and 94% resumed near normal gait. While comparing 2 different routes, the interosseous route or the circum-tibial route, Shah[21] suggested the interosseous route, which yielded a much lower incidence of recurrent inversion deformity of the foot. The circum-tibial route should only be reserved for patients with a calcified and inaccessible interosseous membrane. Furthermore, concomitant tendo Achilles lengthening was also emphasized for equinus deformity.

Reverse Jones Procedure for Dorsal Bunion

Yong, Smith, and Kuo[30] reported a retrospective review of 27 patients (33 feet) who developed a dorsal bunion deformity after previous clubfoot release and had undergone a reverse Jones procedure between 1983 and 2002. There were 18 feet combined with first metatarsal osteotomies and 12 feet with split SPLATTs for better neutralization of the first-ray position and lowering the deforming force from the AT tendon. Before surgery, all patients had a plantar-flexed position of the first metatarsophalangeal joint and obtained an improvement of the lateral metatarsophalangeal angle from the averaged 23° plantar flexion preoperatively to 1° in dorsiflexion postoperatively. The mean global American Orthopedic Foot and Ankle Society hallux metatarsophalangeal-interphalangeal score was 70 preoperatively and increased to 92 postoperatively with improvement on subscores of pain, activity, foot wear, range of motion, callus, and alignment. They concluded that the reverse Jones procedure was an effective means to correct the dorsal bunion deformity, resulting from the muscle imbalance between a weak Achilles tendon and strong flexor hallucis longus.

Peabody Procedure in Myelomeningocele

Individuals with myelomeningocele often present with a calcaneus deformity of the foot as a result of an imbalance between weak or absent plantar-flexor and strong dorsiflexor. This deformity would lead to loss of physiologic toe-off and crouch gait. In dramatic cases, the foot is tipped into more than 40° of dorsiflexion during stance, with ground contact only on the posterior part of the calcaneus. In 1938, Peabody[31] first described the posterior transfer of the AT tendon into the calcaneus to restore plantar flexion in patients with poliomyelitis. The use of ATTT for calcaneal deformity related to myelomeningocele initially received less attention. In 1981, Banta and colleagues[32] reported satisfactory results achieved on 14 feet of 7 patients with myelomeningocele by using combined ATTT and calcaneal tenodesis. In 1991, Fraser and Hoffman[33] reviewed their experience of ATTT and anterior release in 46 feet of 26 patients with myelomeningocele. They reported 89% who had satisfactory results. Besides, they described the neurologic level was an important factor related to the effectiveness of surgery and observed that hip abductor power was a good predictor of a functional transfer. However, a high incidence of secondary deformities after ATTT was also noticed. Valgus deformity commonly resulted (76%) in their series. There was no consensus on the cause of developing this secondary deformity and appropriate solutions.

SUMMARY

Foot and ankle deformities in children can commonly be treated with appropriate soft tissue releases, fusion, or osteotomies to achieve correction. Tendon transfers are useful to achieve and maintain a balanced position of the foot. The procedure is useful to improve foot function for load acceptance, progression of the body over the plantigrade foot during the stance phase of the gait, push-off, and swing phase foot positioning for clearance and initial contact. The authors described 4 tendon transfers useful in the treatment of dynamic foot deformities in children.

REFERENCES

1. Wu KW, Huang SC, Kuo KN, et al. The use of the bio-absorbable screw in a split anterior tibial tendon transfer: a preliminary result. J Pediatr Orthop B 2009;18: 69–72.
2. Garceau GJ. Anterior tibial tendon transposition in recurrent congenital club-foot. J Bone Joint Surg Am 1940;22:932.
3. Laaveg SJ, Ponseti IV. Long-term results of treatment of congenital clubfoot. J Bone Joint Surg Am 1980;62:23–31.
4. Hoffer MM, Reiswig JA, Garret AM, et al. The split anterior tibial tendon transfer in treatment of spastic varus hindfoot of childhood. Orthop Clin North Am 1974;5: 31–8.
5. Kuo KN, Hannigan SP, Hastings ME. Anterior tibial tendon transfer in residual dynamic clubfoot deformity. J Pediatr Orthop 2001;21:35–41.
6. Lapidus PW. Dorsal bunion: its mechanics and operative correction. J Bone Joint Surg Am 1940;22:627–37.
7. Kuo KN. "Reverse Jones" procedure for dorsal bunion following clubfoot surgery. In: Simons GW, editor. The Clubfoot, the present and a view of the future. New York: Springer-Verlag; 1993. p. 384.
8. Thompson GH, Hoyen HA, Barthel T. Tibialis anterior tendon transfer after clubfoot surgery. Clin Orthop Relat Res 2009;467:1306–13.
9. Hoffer MM, Barakat G, Koffman M. Ten year follow-up of split anterior tibial tendon transfer in cerebral palsied patients with spastic equinovarus deformity. J Pediatr Orthop 1985;5:432–4.
10. Krzak JJ, Corcos DM, Graf A, et al. Effect of fine wire electrode insertion on gait patterns in children with hemiplegic cerebral palsy. Gait Posture 2013;37(2): 251–7.
11. Barnes MJ, Herring JA. Combined split anterior tibial-tendon transfer and intramuscular lengthening of the posterior tibial tendon. Results in patients who have a varus deformity of the foot due to spastic cerebral palsy. J Bone Joint Surg Am 1991;73:734–8.
12. Chang CH, Albarracin JP, Lipton GE, et al. Long-term follow-up of surgery for equinovarus foot deformity in children with cerebral palsy. J Pediatr Orthop 2002;22:792–9.

13. Perry J, Waters R, Perrin T. Electromyographic analysis of equinovarus following stroke. Clin Orthop Relat Res 1978;131:47–53.
14. Vogt JC. Split anterior tibial transfer of spastic equinovarus foot deformity. J Foot Ankle Surg 1998;37:1–7.
15. Carda S, Bertoni M, Zerbinati P, et al. Gait change after tendon functional surgery for equinovarus foot in patients with stroke. Am J Phys Med Rehabil 2009;88: 292–301.
16. Hosalkar H, Goebel J, Reddy S, et al. Fixation techniques for split anterior tibialis transfer in spastic equinovarus feet. Clin Orthop Relat Res 2008;466:2500–6.
17. Keenan MA. The management of spastic equinovarus deformity following stroke and head injury. Foot Ankle Clin N Am 2011;16:499–514.
18. Ozkan T, Tuncer S, Ozturk K. Surgical restoration of drop foot deformity with tibialis posterior tendon transfer. Acta Orthop Traumatol Turc 2007;41:259–65.
19. Ozkan T, Tuncer S, Ozturk K. Tibialis posterior tendon transfer for persistent drop foot after peroneal nerve repair. J Reconstr Microsurg 2009;25:157–64.
20. Dreher T, Wolf SI, Heitzmann D, et al. Tibialis posterior tendon transfer corrects the foot drop component of cavovarus foot deformity in Charcot-Marie-Tooth disease. J Bone Joint Surg Am 2014;96:456–62.
21. Shah RK. Tibialis posterior transfer by interosseous route for the correction of foot drop in leprosy. Int Orthop 2009;33:1637–40.
22. Miller GM, Hsu JD, Hoffer MM, et al. Posterior tibial tendon transfer: a review of the literature and analysis of 74 procedures. J Pediatr Orthop 1982;2:363–70.
23. Mayer L. The physiological method of tendon transplantation in the treatment of paralytic drop-foot. J Bone Joint Surg Am 1937;19:389–94.
24. Watkins MB, Jones JB, Ryder CT Jr, et al. Transplantation of the posterior tibial tendon. J Bone Joint Surg Am 1954;36:1181–9.
25. Lipscomb PR, Sanchez JJ. Anterior transplantation of the posterior tibial tendon for persistent palsy of the common peroneal nerve. J Bone Joint Surg Am 1961; 43:60–6.
26. Srinivasan H, Mukherjee SM, Subramaniam RA. Two-tailed transfer of tibialis posterior for correction of drop-foot in leprosy. J Bone Joint Surg Br 1968;50:623–8.
27. Hsu JD, Hoffer MM. Posterior tibial tendon transfer anteriorly through the interosseous membrane: a modification of the technique. Clin Orthop Relat Res 1978; 131:202–4.
28. McCall RE, Frederick HA, McCluskey GM, et al. The Bridle procedure: a new treatment for equines and equinovarus deformities in children. J Pediatr Orthop 1991;11:83–9.
29. Moonot P, Ashwood N, Lockwood D. Orthopaedic complications of leprosy. J Bone Joing Surg Br 2006;87:1328–32.
30. Yong SM, Smith PA, Kuo KN. Dorsal bunion following clubfoot surgery: outcome of reverse Jones procedure. J Pediatr Orthop 2007;27:814–20.
31. Peabody C. Tendon transposition. J Bone Joint Surg Am 1938;20:193–205.
32. Banta JV, Sutherland DH, Wyatt M. Anterior tibial transfer to the os calcis with Achilles tenodesis for calcaneal deformity in myelomeningocele. J Pediatr Orthop 1981;1:125–30.
33. Fraser RK, Hoffman EB. Calcaneus deformity in the ambulant patient with myelomeningocele. J Bone Joing Surg Br 1991;73:994–7.

Syndromic Feet

Arthrogryposis and Myelomeningocele

Harold Jacob Pieter van Bosse, MD

KEYWORDS

- Arthrogryposis multiplex congenita • Myelomeningocele • Spina bifida • Clubfoot
- Calcaneus • Congenital vertical talus • Syndromic foot

KEY POINTS

- Myelomeningocele foot deformities can be congenital (clubfoot, congenital vertical tali), acquired (calcaneus, calcaneovalgus), or a combination (equinus).
- The type of myelomeningocele foot deformity seen is associated with the functional spinal level.
- Clubfeet of myelomeningocele or arthrogrypotic origin have a high recurrence rate, especially with surgical procedures, including soft tissue releases and talectomy.
- Calcaneus and calcaneovalgus foot deformities are best treated early with ongoing bracing to prevent regression and to decrease the number of late presenting deformities.
- Arthrogrypotic foot deformities are the clubfoot and its equinocavus variant, and the congenital vertical talus.

INTRODUCTION

Many of the congenital and developmental idiopathic foot deformities commonly seen also present in children with syndromic conditions. These foot deformities include talipes equino varus (clubfoot) and congenital vertical talus deformities as well as pes planus. The differences between the idiopathic deformities and their syndromic counterparts often related to how early in utero the deformity began to take shape, the subsequent non-pliability of the soft tissues, and the muscle imbalances that induced or maintained the deformity. The range of syndromes that include pediatric foot deformities is vast; this article focuses on only 2 conditions: myelomeningocele and arthrogryposis multiplex congenital. The foot deformities of these 2 conditions are often discussed together, especially clubfoot. Although there are similarities, such as the increased rigidity of the deformities in comparison to idiopathic feet, and imbalances or absence of muscle function, there are also important differences between these similarly appearing feet.

Disclosure Statement: The author has nothing to disclose.
Department of Orthopaedic Surgery, Shriners Hospital for Children, 3551 North Broad Street, Philadelphia, PA 19140, USA
E-mail address: HvanBosse@Shrinenet.org

Foot Ankle Clin N Am 20 (2015) 619–644
http://dx.doi.org/10.1016/j.fcl.2015.07.010
1083-7515/15/$ – see front matter © 2015 Elsevier Inc. All rights reserved.

foot.theclinics.com

MYELOMENINGOCELE

Although the incidence of myelomeningocele has decreased in recent years (1.9/ 10,000 births), it is still the cause for chronic disability in 70,000 to 100,000 persons in the United States,[1,2] with approximately 1500 pregnancies per year affected.[3] The associated foot deformities are particularly difficult to manage, because of the combination of motor paralysis/spasticity and sensory loss. Before the 1950s, the survival rate of afflicted children was low, and those that survived were severely mentally disabled, nonambulatory, and confined to a wheelchair.[4] With the implementation of urgent closure of the spinal defect and techniques to control the hydrocephalus, many if not most of these children will become at least therapeutically ambulatory; those with lower level spinal lesions, with proper care, will continue to be community ambulators in adulthood.[1,2,5–7]

Foot deformities in myelomeningocele can be either congenital or developmental, and the specific deformity that occurs depends to a great extent on the functional neurologic level of involvement.[2,6,8–11] Deformities can be secondary to functional muscles lacking innervated antagonists; denervated muscles reacting spastically rather than flaccidly, due to an intact reflex arc without otherwise intact spinal pathways; or acquired deformities resulting from the cumulative effects of weight-bearing across an unbalanced joint. Although there is considerable overlap, the deformities largely stratify along levels of neurologic involvement.

- In the high-level lesions, thoracic or high lumbar (L1 or L2), a flail foot without deformity and an equinus foot are the most commonly reported.[6,8,9,11] Some of those with equinus, if aggressively treated, can progress to an iatrogenic calcaneus deformity.[6]
- The clubfoot is the most common deformity in infants with midlumbar lesions (L3 and L4)[2,6] and is the most common foot deformity in myelomeningocele overall, present in 30% to 50% of patients.[5,11–13]
- In the low-level lesions (L5 and sacral level), calcaneus deformities or neurologically normal-appearing feet without deformity are present.[6,9,11,14]
- The most common developmental deformity, usually due to years of weight-bearing, is a valgus ankle or pes planovalgus. Most investigators note this as occurring in the lower level lesions,[6,15–17] but some have found this deformity to regularly develop in L3 level lesions as well.[18,19]
- The incidence of vertical tali is about 10%.[20] Sharrard[10] noted that most were congenital, but that some were also developmental, secondary to weight-bearing, with innervation down to at least the L5 or S1 level.[11]

Treatment Considerations

The goal of treating foot deformities in myelomeningocele is very similar to treating all neuromuscular foot deformities: a plantargrade, supple foot that can be comfortably and safely braced, taking into account insensate skin.

- Procedures that stiffen the foot should be avoided, because they make it more difficult to avoid loading pressure points on the skin, which can lead to ulceration.[21–23]
- Cast correction is an important treatment option for most of the foot deformities,[24,25] but the casts must be well padded, pressure points must be avoided, and the casts must be changed relatively frequently to detect skin injury early.
- Most deformities, once corrected, will need constant bracing. Those feet without deformity should be braced to prevent acquired deformity. Other than those with

the lowest spinal level involvement, most patients will require braces for ambulation, or at least will walk more efficiently with braces[26–28]; therefore, instituting brace wear early can help prepare the family and the child for continued wear into late childhood or adulthood.

- In discussing individual studies, we will define a procedure as successful if it results in a plantargrade and braceable foot, requiring no further surgical intervention.

Equinus Foot Deformity

The equinus deformities usually occur in patients with no muscle activity below the knee and are therefore acquired either from the unopposed effects of gravity or from spastic activity of the triceps surae.[2,8,10] Treatment includes regular stretching as well as bracing of flaccid and equinus feet, starting at birth.[11] Should the hindfoot contracture not respond, gentle serial casting, with or without a percutaneous Achilles tenotomy, will likely be sufficient. Achilles tendon resection or a posterior release may be necessary in refractory cases.[2,11]

Talipes Equinovarus (Clubfoot)

The clubfoot is the most common foot deformity in myelomeningocele and is one of the most difficult to treat. Although it can be found at any level of spinal lesion, Sharrard[10] noted that the most severe presentations were those of an L4 level with accompanied spasticity (reflex activity) of lower sacral levels.[11] A study on cadaveric clubfeet of 18- to 20-week-old aborted myelomeningocele fetuses with thoracic/upper lumbar spinal lesions showed that the gastroc soleus was the least affected muscle (least fibrosis), followed by the tibialis anterior and posterior muscles; the peroneus longus had the most fibrosis.[29] This finding would suggest that in high-level myelomeningocele, spastic activity of the triceps surae and both tibialis muscles can cause them to become deforming forces of the foot. Relapse rates of myelomeningocele clubfeet are high, regardless of the treatment method (22%–68%)[10–12,25,30–33]; therefore, treatment should be directed toward modalities that have the best promise of correction without causing irreversible changes to the structure of the foot, which could then limit options for secondary correction after relapse.

Soft tissue release

The traditional treatment approach is the posterior-medial clubfoot release, usually including complete tenotomies or excisions of tendons, rather than lengthenings.[2,11–13] In the series by Sharrard and Grosfield[11] of 54 myelomeningocele patients with 78 clubfeet, corrected with an "extensive medial release," 42 revision procedures were required (46% success rate). Seven of the 54 patients developed skin breakdown of the foot, and another 5 progressed to superficial infection, despite the use of a V-Y incision. Akbar and colleagues[5] reviewed 167 equinovarus deformities corrected by extensive subtalar circumferential releases in 123 patients with myelomeningocele; the age at surgery and follow-up length were not given. They reported 83% success. Muscular imbalance greatly affected success rates, with the highest success rates in the high- or low-level lesions (95% success for thoracic to L2 level, 83% for L5 to sacral level), and the least success for the midlumbar level lesions (64%). de Carvalho Neto and colleagues[12] performed a "radical posteromedial release" with excision of tendons, through a Cincinnati incision.[34] In 63 feet, with an average follow-up of 86 months, the success rate was 63%. Flynn and colleagues[13] reported on 72 feet with 8 years of follow-up that had undergone a radical release. Subsequent procedures, including repeat releases, talectomies, osteotomies, and arthrodesis, were required in 26 feet (success rate of 67%). Bassett and colleagues[35] attempted to avoid skin closure issues by use of soft tissue expanders before the clubfoot release. Two of their 5 patients had myelomeningocele, one of which generated sufficient skin for an excellent skin closure after a complete release; the other developed a severe multiorganism sepsis. The investigators concluded that, in general, soft tissue expansion had limited usefulness before clubfoot surgery.

Talectomy

The excision of the talus is often discussed as either a salvage or a secondary procedure for paralytic clubfoot, creating sufficient laxity to correct both equinus and heel varus deformities without tension.[11,36] There are few studies wherein the specific outcomes for myelomeningocele clubfoot after talectomy are given, but successful outcomes for those studies range between 47% and 75%.[33,37–39] Sherk and Ames[38] reported on 11 children with myelomeningocele who underwent 20 talectomies for clubfoot deformities, at an average of 5.3 years of age. Their longest follow-up was only 5 years, and they noted a 25% rate of deformity recurrence complicating brace wear. In a subsequent follow-up study, Sherk and colleagues,[39] evaluated 19 myelomeningocele patients who underwent 31 talectomies between the ages of 4 and 39 years, with an average follow-up of 12 years. They noted that all feet were corrected enough for shoe wear, but 10% became cavovarus deformities, and 45% had relapses of equinus and varus. Overall, 52% of feet appeared plantargrade, but force plates analysis revealed that only 16% were actually biomechanically plantargrade with uniformly distributed ground reaction forces. Sharrard and Grosfield[11] provided no data on their series, but were among the first to mention that talectomies only could correct hindfoot deformities, and forefoot deformities would require subsequent additional procedures. Similarly, Trumble and colleagues[33] noted only 47% successful results for talectomies performed for 17 myelomeningocele clubfeet at an average age of 3.5 years and an average 7-year follow-up. Failures were primarily due to residual forefoot adductus and supination. Studies on talectomies that grouped multiple diagnoses together are more difficult to interpret. Menelaus[36] included 14 myelomeningocele clubfeet in his series of 41 talectomies, all performed at an average age of 3 years, but as young as 5 months. Their short follow-up (only up to 4 years) yielded a 21% rate of equinus recurrence, with or without varus. Twenty-three of the 28 clubfoot talectomies performed by Dias and Stern[30] were for myelomeningocele. Surgery was performed at an average age of 4.5 years, with an average 4-year follow-up. The overall success rate was only 72%, with failures attributed to residual forefoot deformities.

Two studies with 20-year follow-up, both with mixed diagnoses, had differing outcomes. The series by Cooper and Capello[40] of 26 talectomies included 6 myelomeningocele clubfeet, along with 10 poliomyelitis calcaneo or equinovalgus deformities (and one "no preoperative deformity" foot). The reported success rate was 92%, despite calcaneotibial joint degenerative changes and bony ankylosis observed in many of the older patients. The average patient was 10 years old at the time of surgery, although the investigators stated that the age at surgery was not important. They recommended that this drastic procedure be used only for rigid and severe foot deformities in patients too young for a triple arthrodesis. Legaspi and colleagues[41] had 2 myelomeningocele clubfeet in their study of 24 talectomies. Because of residual hindfoot deformity, the success rate was only 33%. The investigators pointedly did not consider forefoot deformity in their report. Nearly two-thirds of the feet developed tibiocalcaneal arthritis or spontaneous fusion by 10 years after talectomy.

In general, foot fusions (intentional or inadvertent) in patients with myelomeningocele should be avoided, because of the significant concern for decubiti. Maynard and colleagues[22] reviewed 36 myelomeningocele patients, 7 to 30 years old, and found that plantargrade, flexible myelomeningocele feet had a 0% incidence of ulceration, compared with 25% for nonplantargrade flexible feet, 36% for plantargrade rigid feet, and 100% for nonplantargrade rigid feet. Roach and colleagues[23] reviewed 84 adults with myelomeningocele and found surgeries to maintain a plantargrade foot were helpful, because even those with low-level spinal lesions and good strength had trouble ambulating on deformed feet. However, those with plantargrade feet still had a substantial risk of developing pressure sores, many progressing to deep infections and occasional amputations.

Other surgical procedures

The use of external fixators has been well described for treating clubfoot deformities.[42] However, very few studies have included enough myelomeningocele patients from which to draw any conclusions.[32,43,44] Inasmuch as myelodysplasic clubfeet resemble arthrogrypotic ones, the information on external fixator correction in the arthrogryposis section can be extrapolated with caution to the myelodysplastic clubfoot, in the author's opinion, as a last resort.

In response to the difficult circumstances of limited resources in an economically depressed region, Shingade and colleagues[45] developed a single-stage surgical method. Thirty-four children with myelomeningocele clubfeet underwent a percutaneous Achilles tenotomy, plantar fasciotomy, and a closing dorsolateral wedge osteotomy of the midfoot. At a nearly 5-year follow-up, 81% of the feet were rated as good or excellent, using the International Clubfoot Study Group scoring system,[46] although no reference was made as to subsequent operative procedures or neuropathic foot ulceration.

Serial casting

Many investigators have warned about attempting to correct equinovarus foot deformities by serial casting infants or children with myelomeningocele.[5,11] The concerns relate primarily to skin injury secondary to pressure sores. However, as far back as 1971, Walker[47] described the early results of a method of foot manipulation and strapping for newborns with myelomeningocele clubfeet, reminiscent of the "French functional physical therapy method" currently favored at some centers.[48] Of the 35 feet described, 26% were corrected by the strapping, with or without an Achilles tenotomy, and another 60% required a posterior release. Although no indication of length of follow-up was given, the study indicated that these feet could be corrected by largely nonsurgical means. More recently, the Ponseti method[49,50] has emerged as the treatment of choice for not only idiopathic clubfeet but also nonidiopathic clubfeet, including those secondary to myelomeningocele.[25,31,51,52] Gerlach and colleagues[25] prospectively followed a group of 28 clubfeet in 16 patients with myelomeningocele treated with the Ponseti method starting at an average age of 12 weeks, comparing their outcomes to a similarly treated control group of idiopathic clubfeet, with 34 and 37 months average follow-up, respectively. Correction was obtained in 27 of the 28 feet, requiring the same number of casts for correction as the idiopathic clubfeet. The correction was maintained with a foot abduction orthosis, either the standard static or the dynamic kind. Relapse developed in 68% of the myelomeningocele feet compared with 26% of the idiopathic feet; 79% of the myelomeningocele relapses were successfully treated with repeat casting, although 4 feet required extensive soft tissue release. Janicki and colleagues[31] reported on a similar study including 9 myelomeningocele clubfeet, all of which were initially corrected by the Ponseti method starting at an average of 11 weeks of age. Afterward, they were maintained in a static foot abduction orthosis. At a mean follow-up of 33 months, 44% of the myelomeningocele feet remained corrected, 22% had a relapse that responded to repeat casting, but another 33% required surgical releases to correct their relapse. Gurnett and colleagues[51] also evaluated outcomes of 84 Ponseti treated nonidiopathic clubfeet, 17 of which were myelomeningocele clubfeet. The results were not parsed by specific diagnosis, but the investigators noted that the nonidiopathic clubfeet required on average one more cast for correction compared with the idiopathic feet. At a minimum of 2-year follow-up, the nonidiopathic clubfeet had a 15% relapse rate compared with 4%, most of which responded to repeat casting.

Author's preference
The author is a strong proponent of the Ponseti method for treatment of nonidiopathic clubfeet. The rate of relapse of the myelomeningocele clubfoot, regardless of treatment, is high. Unfortunately, if the initial correction is surgical, most surgeons continue that course for subsequent relapses, with ever more damaging effects. A posteromedial release will lead to a stiffened foot, which will be more difficult to treat after relapse, but the author has had good success regaining correction with serial casting. Talectomies fundamentally alter the structure of the foot, making it more difficult to recover from a relapse, truly a "burned bridge." Similarly, Grice or triple arthrodeses may acutely achieve a desired correction, but any relapse can only be treated with extensive surgery, and even if the foot shape is maintained, the risk for pressure sores is high. The author thinks the best strategy is to obtain correction of the clubfoot deformity with the Ponseti method and then maintain it with a well-molded ankle-foot orthosis (AFO), one that is molded to correct the heel varus and forefoot adductus (**Fig. 1**). The anterior ankle strap originates inside the brace on the lateral side, to help roll the ankle out of varus. Medial and lateral straps from the footplate to the upper brace region act as dorsiflexion straps at nighttime. Relapses should be treated with repeat casting. For feet that are particularly challenging, delaying surgical correction until 10 to 12 years of age has a higher likelihood of success, because there is less prospective growth remaining. In the event of a severely rigid deformity, but without bony ankylosis, a soft tissue Ilizarov frame may be effective, essentially applying an external fixator to the foot, without soft tissue releases or osteotomies, with the goal to correct the foot similarly to the Ponseti method of abduction stretching.[53–56]

Calcaneus Foot Deformity
The calcaneus deformity in myelomeningocele is caused by unopposed action of the ankle dorsiflexors, either volitional or spastic, relative to weak or absent ankle plantarflexors. The peroneus brevis may dislocate from its groove behind the lateral malleolus, becoming an ankle dorsiflexor and evertor; the tibialis anterior may subluxate laterally, paradoxically everting the foot as well.[10] The deformity occurs most often in those with L4 or L5 level of involvement, affecting 17% to 35% of patients with myelomeningocele.[5,6,20,57,58] The gait characteristics are loss of the normal toe-off, and a progressive crouch gait until static forces prevent further ankle dorsiflexion, leading to a prolonged knee extensor moment during stance.[59] If uncorrected, heel ulceration may develop, leading to osteomyelitis (**Fig. 2**).

There is a rich body of literature dedicated exclusively to the treatment of the calcaneus foot deformity in children with myelomeningocele. Early surgical intervention to prevent the development of a more rigid deformity is recommended by most investigators,[57,58,60] especially because prolonged weight-bearing may lead to calcaneovalgus deformities and external tibial torsion.[58,61,62] Tendon transfers to substitute for the absent or poor ankle plantarflexion power are the most commonly described

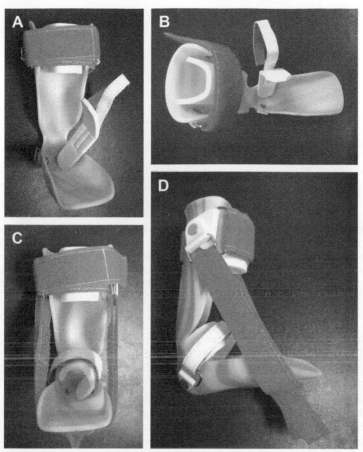

Fig. 1. Left dual purpose AFO molded for correction of hindfoot varus and forefoot adductus, the anterior ankle strap originating in the inner lateral aspect of the brace. (*A*) Perspective from directly anterior, demonstrating the origin of the anterior ankle strap. (*B*) View from a superior perspective shows straight medial border. (*C*) Anterior perspective with removable dorsiflexion straps in place. (*D*) Medial view with dorsiflexion straps applied.

procedures, usually a transfer of the anterior tibialis posteriorly through the interosseous membrane to the calcaneal tuberosity.[10,11,57,58,60,63–66] Results of this procedure have been variable, though, with both limited success, as well as cases of weak or nonfunctioning tendon transfers or severe deformity development. Bliss and Menelaus[60] reviewed 25 patients who had undergone 46 anterior tibialis transfers for calcaneus deformity as children, with an average follow-up age of 22 years. Only 10 transfers were plantargrade or in mild and acceptable equinus at follow-up; the others reverted to calcaneus or overcorrected to equinus deformities, regardless of whether the transfers were functioning or not. Sixty-six additional procedures were required for 36 feet, which, using the definition of success (a plantargrade and braceable foot, requiring no further surgical intervention), yielded a 22% success rate. Janda and colleagues[66] reviewed 12 feet of 6 patients who had undergone transfers and found that 50% of the feet had nonfunctioning transfers; yet these 6 feet were plantargrade. Paradoxically, of the 6 functioning transfers, 5 developed secondary deformities

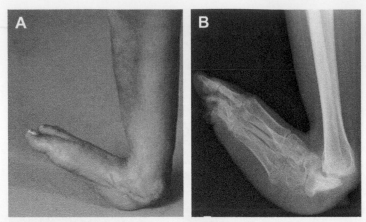

Fig. 2. Right foot with calcaneus deformity of a 15-year-old girl with L4 level myelomeningocele. The foot initially presented as a clubfoot, and she was treated with bilateral talectomies. The patient has ambulated chronically on the heel, leading to several episodes of severe decubiti and osteotomyelitis. (A) Clinical view of the medial foot, weight-bearing. (B) Radiographic view of the same foot. Note the absence of the talus and the loss of the calcaneal tuberosity and body, probably due to debridement for osteomyelitis.

(planovalgus, equinovalgus, equinovarus), 3 requiring surgical correction (success rate of 58%). Fraser and Hoffman[14] reported on 46 feet in 26 patients who had undergone the transfer, with 64% having the ability to stand on their toes. Their results were tempered by the development of secondary deformities in 76% of the feet; 33 of the 46 feet required subsequent operations for an actual success rate of 28%. Several studies suggested that the anterior tibialis tendon to calcaneus transfer was more likely to be nonfunctional if performed before 4 or 5 years of age, possibly because it is difficult to assess before that age if a child has volitional control over the muscle.[60,63,64,66,67]

From the discussion above, it can be seen that success or failure was not well associated with a functioning or nonfunctioning transfer. Dynamic studies may help explain this inconsistency. Banta and colleagues[63] and Stott and colleagues[67] both noted a pattern of continuous anterior tibialis activity on dynamic electromyography, both in swing and in stance phases. Janda and colleagues[66] found 3 patterns of muscle activity in gait: during the stance phase alone, during the swing phase alone, and a pattern of continuous of activity similar to what the other investigators had identified. The continuous pattern likely represented a spastic muscle, in which case it would be better to transect the tendon rather than transfer it.[63,67] Although these gait studies did show that the calcaneus deformity did not progress, the transfers could not prevent excessive ankle dorsiflexion in stance; the investigators all recommended continued usage of postoperative orthotic support.[63,66,67]

One criticism of the posterior transfer of the anterior tibialis tendon is that the muscle simply is not strong enough to substitute for the triceps surae. In fact, the combined power of all the ankle muscles is still less than the power of the triceps surae.[68] Wenz and colleagues[69] not only transferred 6 tendons (tibialis anterior and posterior, peroneus brevis and longus, extensor digitorum and hallucis longus) to the Achilles but also performed an inverse Lambrinudi, essentially a triple arthrodesis, which also elevates the profile of the talus to function as a bone block against the anterior distal tibia, limiting dorsiflexion. Nine patients, average age 17.5 years, were evaluated at an average of 32 months postoperatively. All but one could ambulate without AFOs. The investigators did note that 2 patients required anterior transfer of the long toe flexor tendons for disabling foot drop. Furthermore, the follow-up was too short to determine the risk for degenerative ankle changes from the bone block impinging on the distal tibia. Others have found success with lesser adjunct procedures. Georgiadis and Aronson[64] noted that 12 of their 39 feet required other procedures after the anterior tibialis tendon transfer to the calcaneus, for an initial success rate of 72%. Those 12 feet underwent subsequent tendinous procedures (releases or transfers) and/or subtalar/triple arthrodeses to correct residual deformities, for a success rate at 6-year follow-up of 95%. Park and colleagues[57] performed anterior tibialis tendon transfers on 31 calcaneus feet at an average age of 7 years, 12 patients having concomitant osseous procedures to balance their feet. These ancillary procedures included supramalleolar procedures to correct ankle positioning (varus, valgus, or rotational), calcaneal lengthening osteotomies, and subtalar arthrodeses. They noted no deformity recurrence or progression, or development of secondary deformities at a mean follow-up of 47 months for a 100% success rate.

Another treatment strategy for the calcaneus foot is a complete anterolateral release of the ankle. Rodrigues and Dias[58] included sectioning the ankle dorsiflexors and toe extensors as well as the peroneus brevis and longus as part of their release. Of their 76 patients, 62 had a plantargrade and braceable foot, for an 82% success rate. Of the 14 that failed, 6 required a repeat procedure, and 8 underwent Achilles release for equinus deformity. Swaroop and Dias[2] suggested that long-standing rigid deformities could be addressed with an anterolateral release, combined with a posteriorly based closing wedge osteotomy of the calcaneal tuberosity to shift the tuberosity more posterior and proximal. These procedures have been described primarily for patients with polio, so extrapolation to myelomeningocele calcaneus feet is intriguing but untested.[70,71]

Author's preference

Casting and bracing should be the hallmarks to prevention of a severe calcaneus foot deformity. In cases of established deformity, surgical correction is required with attention to eliminating deforming forces, possibly augmenting the ankle plantarflexors, and balancing the foot with bony and tendinous procedures. The anterior tibialis tendon transfer to the calcaneus is a tempting procedure, because it both removes a deforming force and augments ankle plantarflexion strength, but care should be taken not to transfer a spastic tendon. If the tendon is transferred, other procedures to balance the foot may be necessary in roughly 50% of cases. As discussed early in this article, fusions should be avoided, because they can lead to increased skin loading pressures and decubiti. Equinus deformity should be prevented by not overtensioning the transfer and by postoperative bracing. Patients should expect to be braced chronically postoperatively. If tendon transfer is not possible, other procedures such as anterior ankle release are more ablative but may be beneficial. Preoperative casting has been beneficial to decrease the severity of a deformity.

Valgus Hindfoot and Ankle Deformities

Valgus deformities of the hindfoot and ankle region must be assessed carefully in order to determine if the deformity is supratalar or infratalar or both. The literature provides many examples of corrective procedure for the valgus foot having failed because of a missed valgus ankle deformity.[16,17] The valgus deformities occur primarily in weight-bearing patients and develop over time[61,62]; Frischhut and colleagues[6] noted no such deformities at 2 years of age, but by 10 years, approximately 20% of

L3-L4 patients and 45% of L5-sacral patients displayed the finding. This percentage further increased to 55% in the latter group by 25 years of age.

Valgus hindfoot correction

Swaroop and Dias[2] recommend treating the isolated heel valgus with a reverse Koutsogiannis osteotomy,[72] essentially a bone cut perpendicular to the axis of the calcaneal tuberosity just anterior to the insertion of the Achilles. The tuberosity is then shifted medially, to position it in line with the ankle. Foot abduction can be corrected with an opening wedge cuboid osteotomy.[2] Torosian and Dias[17] reported 82% good results in 38 feet treated in this manner, at greater than 5-year follow-up. Three of the poor results were due to unrecognized ankle valgus. The advantage of the procedure is that no joints are violated, and therefore, there is less risk of stiffness. Other investigators have suggested arthrodeses to gain correction.[73] In a study of 14 myelomeningocele feet having undergone subtalar arthrodeses at an average age of 6 years, Gallien and colleagues[74] found only a 61% success rate at an average follow-up of 4 years, due to residual valgus deformity or the development of a varus hindfoot. Aronson and Middleton[75] reviewed the outcomes of 20 feet an average of 4 years after extra-articular subtalar arthrodeses. The patients were an average of 7 years old at the time of surgery. Satisfactory results were noted in 90% of cases, and the 2 unsatisfactory cases were due to residual ankle valgus. Despite the good outcome, significant concerns remain related to the association of diminishing foot flexibility and skin ulceration in myelomeningocele as these children age into adults.[22]

Etiology of the valgus ankle

According to Dias,[62] the valgus ankle develops in patients with L5 or higher functional levels, where the weakened soleus muscle exerts less of a downwards pull on the fibula.[62] As a result, there is less growth stimulation of the distal fibula, and a gradual relative shortening of the lateral malleolus. Altered compression forces at the ankle and inhibition of growth of the distal lateral tibial physis occur, resulting in the development of distal tibial epiphyseal wedging. The explanation favored by this author is that the foot, due to weakened or absent ankle stabilizing musculature, rolls into maximum valgus until soft tissue or bony constraints block further motion, much as the calcaneus foot can only dorsiflex so far until the posterior soft tissue structures of the ankle or anterior ankle impingement limit further collapse. With continued weight-bearing, force is concentrated on the lateral distal tibial plafond and the lateral malleolus, which causes a growth inhibition consistent with the Heuter-Volkmann law.[76]

Fibular-Achilles tendodesis

Westin[77] began treating pes calcaneus deformities in polio patients with a tenodesis of the Achilles to the tibia. In one case, he unintentionally sutured the Achilles to the fibula, and over 18 months the fibula was observed to hypertrophy and lengthen. Although Westin and colleagues[78] initially thought the procedure was contraindicated in myelomeningocele, others have found it beneficial. Fucs and colleagues[15] described the outcomes of the procedure on 17 calcaneovalgus feet in 11 patients with myelomeningocele, along with 8 poliomyelitis feet; average age at surgery was 8.5 years with a mean 6.5 years of follow-up. Concurrent procedures were performed to correct the foot deformity or balance the foot. All feet were reportedly plantargrade, but the success rate was 76% due to a high rate of secondary procedures, primarily to correct residual pes planus. Stevens and Toomey[79] reported on 32 ankles in 18 patients, who also underwent a fibular-Achilles tenodesis. Surgery was performed at a mean of 6 years, with follow-up of nearly 3 years. Four patients had simultaneous subtalar fusions to correct hindfoot valgus. Six ankles failed to improve, for a success rate of 81%. Seven subsequent derotational osteotomies needed to be done for pre-existing external torsion of the tibia. This author wonders if the Achilles tenodesis is more effective when done to the fibula rather than to the tibia is because the fibula is more posterior, and therefore, represents a more perpendicular vector to the motion of the calcaneal tuberosity when the foot is near plantargrade. In fact, the direction of the tenodesed tendon is similar to the intact Achilles tendon.

Hemiepiphysiodesis of the medial distal tibia
In growing children with a mild ankle valgus and a triangular-shaped distal tibial physis, a medial distal tibial hemi-epiphysiodesis can allow for gradual correction of the deformity. Burkus and colleagues[19] described the procedure with use of staples on 12 patients with myelomeningocele at an average age of 10.5 years. The tibiotalar joint averaged 10° of valgus preoperatively, which was corrected to 6° of varus on average. At physeal closure, all patients maintained their corrections. Stevens and Belle[80] had a similar series, but with a more heterogeneous group of diagnoses; only 5 of 31 patients with ankle valgus had myelomeningocele, and the results were not diagnosis specific. The epiphysiodesis was performed with a cannulated 4.5-mm screw through the medial malleolus. All 50 ankles were corrected out of valgus. Five patients actually overcorrected into varus due to negligent follow-up, but no corrective procedures were performed.

Distal tibial osteotomy
In more severe valgus deformities, or in patients with insufficient remaining growth, supramalleolar corrective osteotomies are effective. Sharrard and Webb[81] performed 16 supramalleolar wedge osteotomies on 13 children, with an average age of 9.5 years. Thirteen feet were well corrected, but 2 feet collapsed into valgus and another was overcorrected, all three requiring repeat osteotomies. Abraham and colleagues[18] performed 55 supramalleolar osteotomies in 35 myelomeningocele patients, at an average age of 12 years. The average preoperative tibiatalar valgus was 18°, which was corrected an average of 17°. The investigators noted that the best results were in those slightly overcorrected to 5° of varus. The success rate was 76%, with unsuccessful cases due to loss of correction or nonunion. Lubicky and Altiok[82] described a transphyseal osteotomy of the distal tibia, appropriate for children 9 years or older, because the growth from the contralateral unaffected distal tibial physis would not be sufficient to cause a symptomatic limb length discrepancy. With such a distal osteotomy, the investigators stated, the primary deformity is corrected without creating a compensatory deformity; future deformity is prevented by a simultaneous epiphysiodesis of the distal tibia. Twelve ankles in 9 children with myelomeningocele were treated, with only one patient having more than 5° residual valgus at follow-up.

Author's preference
Many of the foot deformities in myelomeningocele are developmental or at least progressive. Early and active care may help to prevent the deformities that later require extensive surgical attention. In the infants, gentle serial casting will correct the calcaneus deformity in most cases, although a percutaneous tenotomy of a spastic anterior tibialis tendon may be necessary. Then, a well-molded AFO should be issued, with correction of hindfoot valgus and forefoot adductus, an anterior ankle strap starting inside medially to help shift the heel out of valgus, and a well-padded forefoot strap to counter ankle dorsiflexion. Such bracing will help to mitigate the deforming forces of gravity as the child becomes weight-bearing. The braces will also improve the child's gait efficiency and energy consumption.[26–28]

Congenital Vertical Talus

Congenital vertical tali are relatively rare in myelomeningocele, seen in approximately 10% of newborns.[6,10,11,20] Sharrard and Grosfield[11] found that the congenital vertical tali were usually found in patients with an L5 or S1 level lesion and suggested that the preserved action of the foot dorsiflexors and evertors, unopposed by the long toe flexors and foot intrinsics, everted and pronated the forefoot. The talus and calcaneus, held in plantarflexion by the spastic triceps surae, allowed the Chopart joint to become unstable, with the navicular displacing to the dorsum of the neck of the talus.[11] Drennan and Sharrard,[83] in describing the autopsy findings of an infant with myelomeningocele and a vertical talus, suggested that the imbalance between a functioning anterior tibialis and diminished posterior tibialis also had a substantial role.

Several surgical releases have been discussed in the past,[84,85] but the minimally invasive technique developed by Dobbs and colleagues[86,87] is really the most effective and efficient treatment of this deformity. The corrective method features gentle but progressive plantarflexion and adduction stretching of the forefoot, while providing superolaterally directed pressure on the plantarly displaced head of the talus. This position is furthered in subsequent serial cast changes. Once the forefoot deformity is well corrected, surgery is indicated: a small medial incision is used to visualize and reduce the talonavicular joint, which is then stabilized with a Kirschner wire. Chalayon and colleagues[24] described using the procedure on 25 nonidiopathic congenital vertical tali from 15 patients, 4 of whom (6 feet) had myelomeningocele. Casting was initiated at a mean age of 6 months, and follow-up was at a mean age of 3.5 years. All of the myelomeningocele patients were successfully corrected without recurrences. Three of the 4 were community ambulators; the fourth was a household ambulator.

ARTHROGRYPOSIS MULTIPLEX CONGENITA

Arthrogryposis multiplex congenita, or arthrogryposis, is not a diagnosis of itself, but actually a descriptive term for the more than 400 conditions with the shared presentation of an infant born with at least 2 or more joint contractures in multiple body areas.[88,89] Characteristically, these conditions have fetal akinesia in common, where the lack of spontaneous motion can be secondary to nerve or muscle abnormalities, or the development of constricting soft tissue. When a developing joint does not range through its arc of motion, it promotes fibrosis of the normally pliant soft tissues surrounding the joints, which is the genesis of the contractures.[88] Arthrogryposis occurs in approximately 1 of every 3000 live births, with the most common or classic form, amyoplasia, occurring in 1 of every 10,000 births.[88]

There are essentially 3 kinds of arthrogrypotic foot deformities:

- The "classic" clubfoot (**Fig. 3**)
- The equinocavus foot (**Fig. 4**)
- The congenital vertical talus (**Fig. 5**).

The Classic Clubfoot

Clubfeet are the most common foot deformities in arthrogryposis and tend to be more rigid and severe than their idiopathic counterparts.[36,90–93] Early treatment has long been recommended, to make the most of the suppleness of the newborn. Historically, though, treatment has been surgical, with a spectrum of progressively more extensive procedures advocated, as both primary and secondary interventions. The most often described surgeries are soft tissue releases and talectomies.

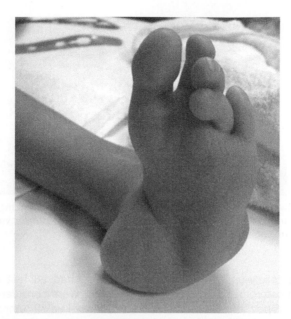

Fig. 3. Classic clubfoot. Note the severe heel varus and adductus.

Soft tissue releases

Soft tissue procedures may be as simple as an Achilles tenotomy, or as elaborate as a radical soft tissue release.[90,91,93–103] Reported satisfactory results range from 100% to 21% for different soft tissue procedures, with the suggestion that better results were obtained by operating at an earlier age with more aggressive procedures. Carlson and colleagues[90] found that 73% of their 41 patients required repeat surgery, averaging 2.5 procedures per foot. Drummond and Cruess[91] reported that only 6 of 23 posterior releases performed at an average age of 2.7 years derived lasting benefit at an

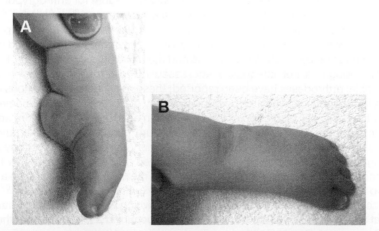

Fig. 4. Equinocavus clubfoot variant. (*A*) Lateral view of the left foot depicting the severe hindfoot equinus and deep transverse cavus. The toes are mildly flexed in this uncorrected foot. (*B*) Dorsal view of the same foot shows relatively mild forefoot adductus.

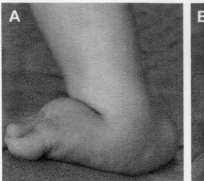
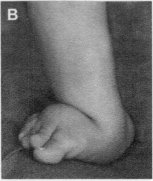

Fig. 5. Congenital vertical talus. (*A*) Lateral view of the right foot, depicting hindfoot equinus with severe forefoot dorsiflexion and mild toe flexion. (*B*) Anterior view of the same foot shows the forefoot abductus.

average 10-year follow-up.[91] Guidera and Drennan[94] had 28 feet in 15 patients that underwent posteromedial releases, but only 25% were considered successful. Södergård and Ryöppy[101] performed soft tissue releases on 52 arthrogrypotic clubfeet, at an average of 3 weeks of age, with a success rate of 48% at a follow-up of 1 to 36 years, compared with 75% success for the 20 feet corrected with casting alone. Niki and colleagues[97] describe the outcomes at a nearly 10-year average follow-up on 41 clubfeet in 22 patients with amyoplasia, who underwent posteromedial releases at an average age of 7.3 months. They noted a 73% relapse rate, of which 8 of 28 feet responded well to serial casting. Menelaus[36] thought that the high rate of relapse after soft tissue releases in arthrogrypotic clubfeet was due to the inability to sufficiently release the contracted medial soft tissues, and the lack of adaptive changes of the medial tarsal bones, which remain wedged apart medially rather than molding to each other.[36]

Talectomy

Talectomies have been regarded as both a primary procedure for arthrogrypotic clubfeet[36,37,91,94,104–106] and a salvage procedure after recurrences.[30,37,41,91,94,104–107] As discussed in the myelomeningocele section on talectomies, the procedure provides laxity in the hindfoot to allow correction of equinus and varus deformities and creates a stable articulation between the calcaneus and the ankle mortise.[36,41,104,105] Forefoot deformity, though, is not adequately addressed by talectomies.[30,41] Spontaneous calcaneotibial arthrodeses have been reported; these may not have as serious consequences for the patients with arthrogryposis as they do for those with myelomeningocele, but they may still lead to point loading on skin and decubiti formation, and late, rigid deformity (**Fig. 6**).[72,105,106,108,109] The literature presents a complex and fragmented picture, because most studies group primary and salvage talectomy procedures together. Solund and colleagues[108] reviewed 14 feet in 8 children who had undergone talectomies as a salvage procedure at a mean age of 8 years; at an average follow-up of 13 years, their success rate was 64%. Green and colleagues[107] had a 56% success rate in 34 feet of 18 patients, half of which were done as a primary talectomy, at an average 11-year follow-up. Relapses occurred 2 to 6 years after the operation. Cassis and Capdevila[104] described results in 16 primary and 85 salvage talectomies done at an average age of 4.3 years, with mean follow-up of 6 years. They reported good results in 65% of cases, which they generously defined as up

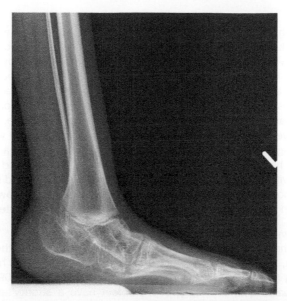

Fig. 6. Lateral radiograph of the left foot of a 10-year-old girl with arthrogryposis and bilateral clubfeet, who at 6 years of age underwent bilateral talectomies. Despite diligent use of braces and intermittent corrective casting, she still developed a rigid 20° equinus and 20° varus hindfoot contracture and was found to have developed a tibiocalcaneal fusion.

to 15° of equinus and adductus. D'Souza and colleagues[110] had an average 11-year follow-up on 11 children with 21 talectomies, 8 of which were the primary procedure. The talectomies were performed at a mean age of 3.5 years, with a satisfactory rate (<10° equinus) of 74%. Some investigators have suggest that talectomies should be the primary procedure for all arthrogrypotic clubfeet, but those investigators base their recommendations on 1 or 2 patients in their studies, with limited documented follow-up.[94,108] Larger series report the satisfactory rate of primary talectomies as only 45% to 50%.[37,91,98,105]

External fixator correction
Franke and colleagues[53] and Grille and Franke[54] published the earliest articles on correcting severe clubfoot deformities with the Ilizarov frame. They relied on soft tissue distraction to facilitate correction, avoiding osteotomies. In their initial article, 1 of their 5 patients had arthrogryposis, with an average age of 11 years. At a 3-year follow-up, all feet were plantargrade, although stiffness of the subtalar and midfoot joints was common.[54] A follow-up article included 4 arthrogrypotic clubfeet, treated similarly. At 5-year follow-up, all feet were plantargrade, and all participants were able to wear normal shoes.[53] El Barbary and colleagues[111] had 23 arthrogrypotic clubfeet treated with soft tissue distraction using an Ilizarov frame, at an average of 8.5 years. At an average of 40 months, all feet were plantargrade, despite mild adductus in a few feet. Brunner and colleagues[112] used the Ilizarov to correct the equinus of 16 arthrogrypotic clubfeet, using soft tissue distraction. The success rate was 63%, with several of the failures requiring talectomies. Ilizarov soft tissue distraction was also used by Choi and colleagues[113] to correct 12 recurrent arthrogrypotic clubfeet, at a mean age of 5 years. At a mean follow-up of 35 months, all but 2 of the feet were plantargrade.

Serial casting

Several studies have demonstrated that the Ponseti method is effective in treating arthrogrypotic clubfeet.[31,114–116] Boehm and colleagues[116] treated 24 clubfeet in 12 infants born with distal arthrogryposis. At a minimum 2-year follow-up, 6 feet had relapsed, of which 4 were corrected with casting and the other 2 required extensive soft tissue releases. Morcuende and colleagues[114] treated 32 clubfeet in 16 patients with arthrogryposis, with an average of 4 years of follow-up. Five patients required extensive soft tissue release, due to either lack of correction or relapse. Janicki and colleagues[31] reviewed a mixed group of nonidiopathic clubfeet treated with the Ponseti method, including 8 arthrogrypotic feet in 5 patients. Two patients had a good result; 2 more patients had bilateral failures requiring surgery, and one had bilateral recurrences treated with casting. van Bosse and colleagues[115] performed Ponseti casting on 10 arthrogrypotic patients (19 feet). At an average 38 months follow-up, 8 feet had relapses, requiring repeat casting. Two patients (4 feet) required posterior releases.

Author's preference

Patients with arthrogryposis constitute approximately 80% of the author's practice. In the past 7 years, approximately 75% of the arthrogryposis patients have undergone clubfoot casting (**Fig. 7**). Since the publication of the series in 2009,[115] the author has come to realize that arthrogrypotic clubfeet have a strong tendency toward relapse, regardless of the method of treatment, and he has moved toward repeatedly casting the relapses, avoiding any intensive procedures for these feet. In doing so, the author has not performed any soft tissue releases more extensive than an Achilles tenotomy nor any talectomies on these children in greater than a decade. The author's practice is to attempt to space out the time between casting series by at least a year, and he finds that as a child grows, relapses become less frequent. The author has developed many modifications on the Ponseti method for these patients.

- In feet with more than 40° equinus, an initial percutaneous Achilles tenotomy is performed just before the first cast or early in the casting series. This tenotomy allows the calcaneus to be unlocked from the back of the tibia; otherwise, it would not be able to swing out of varus.
- In stiffer feet, or in older children, the pressure needed over the lateral head of the talus to counter the abduction forces of stretching and casting would likely cause skin injury. Therefore, in such cases, the practitioner molding the cast should apply the flat of their hand over the anterolateral aspect of the ankle/foot dorsum, to distribute pressure evenly, avoiding pressure over the lateral malleolus. Alternatively, the knee can be held firmly, so that the ankle mortise stabilizes the talus.
- Once correction is obtained, the author uses an AFO, molded to correct heel varus and forefoot adductus, with the anterior ankle strap starting inside laterally, to roll the ankle in to valgus. The braces have medial and lateral dorsiflexion straps to stretch the ankles at nighttime (see **Fig. 1**). Initially, when the author began treating arthrogryposis clubfeet, he used the standard foot abduction orthosis, but was frustrated with the very rapid relapses. It seemed that the arthrogrypotic children do not kick like those with idiopathic clubfeet, which helps to stretch the ankles. Also, the hip and knee contractures often make it impossible to position the foot abduction brace to place the feet in the appropriate amount of external rotation.
- These strategies have worked well, even in those relapses that have been referred following aggressive soft tissue releases or talectomies. The strategies have also been effective in correcting neglected arthrogrypotic clubfeet in older children, well into the teenage years.

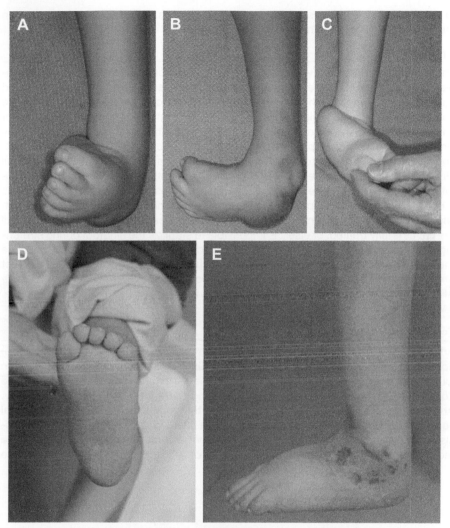

Fig. 7. Correction of a classic clubfoot. A 3-year-old boy with arthrogryposis, adopted to the United States with no previous attention to his clubfeet. (*A*) Anterior view of the left foot demonstrating the severe supination and heel varus, precasting. (*B*) Lateral view of the same foot, with large soft tissue callus from weight-bearing on the uncorrected foot. (*C*) Plantar view of the same foot pretreatment, with moderate forefoot adductus, but also demonstrating the severe hindfoot equinus, which is obscured by the heel varus and forefoot supination. (*D*) Plantar view of the left foot, approximately 1 year after casting. (*E*) Lateral view of the same foot. Correction is maintained with an AFO, including dorsiflexion straps at nighttime.

The "soft tissue Ilizarov frame" has been effective for the occasional older child with a severely rigid deformity, such as a postsurgical relapse or neglected clubfoot, without bony ankylosis. Initial casting may decrease the deformity enough to make frame application less taxing. The author has only used this for children 12 years of age or older, with little growth remaining. Essentially, the external fixator is applied to the foot without soft tissue releases or osteotomies, with subsequent correction mimicking the Ponseti method of abduction stretching.[53–56]

Equinocavus Foot

The equinocavus foot is a variant of the typical clubfoot, but with equinus and complete midfoot cavus as the major deformities; heel varus, forefoot supination, and adductus are relatively minor components. The midfoot crease traverses the entire sole of the foot, from medial to lateral. Toe flexion contractures are usually present and are often very resistant to stretching. The appearance of the foot is strikingly similar to the atypical or complex clubfoot,[117] often including the hammertoe/shortened position of the great toe. The stretching method is similar to that of the atypical clubfoot as well, placing the index and forefingers of both hands on the dorsum of the midfoot, just anterior to the ankle joint, and the thumbs under the metatarsal heads (**Fig. 8**). Gradual upwards pressure on the metatarsal heads, relative to the midfoot, allows for correction of the midfoot cavus (**Fig. 9**). Achilles tenotomies are delayed until the cavus is fully treated, or else it is impossible to stabilize the hindfoot during stretching. The typical Ponseti abduction stretching and casting should be avoided, because the foot will quickly overcorrect, resulting in an ugly equinovalgus foot with a midfoot break that is challenging to reverse. After correction, the author uses the same style AFO. Anecdotally, the equinocavus foot seems to have a lower tendency to relapse, if well braced.

Congenital Vertical Talus

Arthrogrypotic congenital vertical tali have a much lower incidence (3%–10%) compared with arthrogrypotic clubfeet (78%–90%).[89,93] Just as the arthrogrypotic clubfoot is more severe and stiff than its idiopathic counterpart, the arthrogrypotic congenital vertical talus can be more challenging to treat than the idiopathic variety. Aroojis and colleagues[118] reviewed their 26 arthrogrypotic patients with congenital vertical tali and found that none had amyoplasia. Instead, the underlying arthrogryposis conditions included distal arthrogryposis, contractural syndromes, or some of the more severe syndromic or unclassified forms of arthrogryposis. Depending on the

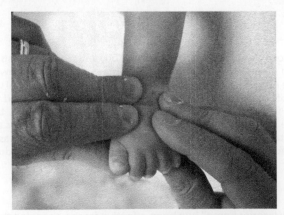

Fig. 8. Hand positioning to correct the equinocavus foot. Known as the 4-finger technique, the index and long fingers of both hands are over the midfoot, acting as a fulcrum for the dorsiflexion pressure over the heads of the metatarsals, applied by the thumbs. The technique relies on counterforce of the Achilles tendon; therefore, an Achilles tenotomy should not be done until after the midfoot cavus is corrected.

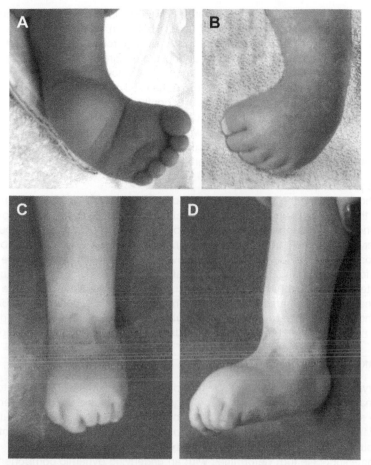

Fig. 9. Correction of an equinocavus foot. (*A*) Plantar view of the left foot of a 2-month-old infant girl, before casting, demonstrating the deep midfoot crease, traversing the entire foot, and the relatively mild heel varus and forefoot adductus. (*B*) View of the foot dorsum of the same foot, pretreatment. The toe flexion contractures can be appreciated. (*C*) Anterior view of the same foot nearly 2 years after casting, with good correction of the forefoot adductus. (*D*) Lateral view of the same foot demonstrating correction of the cavus. The foot could dorsiflex well above neutral. The toe contractures have relapsed and continue to be a problem.

grouping of the underlying arthrogrypotic condition, the investigators found that either the feet could be relatively straightforward to correct using an open one-stage procedure or the feet could be very difficult to correct with a high rate of poor results. Ramanoudjame and colleagues[119] discussed 31 feet in 22 children, 7 with arthrogryposis, who underwent a 2-incision midtarsal surgical release, essentially a complete capsulotomy of the talonavicular and calcaneocuboid joints, along with lengthening of the tibialis anterior, peroneus brevis, extensors digitorum longus, and hallucis longus. Overall good results were 77% at 11-year follow-up, although these were not broken down by diagnosis. Reoperation was necessary in 16%.

The Dobbs method[86,87] for treating the arthrogrypotic congenital vertical tali has proved to be very effective. Wright and colleagues[120] noted that in the nonisolated congenital vertical tali undergoing the Dobbs method of reverse Ponseti casting, all of the feet that were initially treated without an open reduction of the talonavicular joint eventually required one. Comparison of scores between feet with a recurrence and those without showed that the feet with the recurrence fared much more poorly. Therefore, they recommended a mini–open reduction as standard protocol for all nonisolated congenital vertical tali. Chalayon and colleagues[24] described using the procedure on 25 nonidiopathic congenital vertical tali from 15 patients, 5 of whom (9 feet) had arthrogryposis. Casting was initiated at a mean age of 6 months, and follow-up was at a mean age of 3.5 years. All of the patients were successfully corrected, but one of the arthrogrypotic children had a recurrence, which was treated by recasting and then pinning of both the talonavicular and the calcaneocuboid joints. Three of the 5 cases were community ambulators; the other 2 cases were household ambulators.

Author's preference

The author has found the Dobbs method to be unquestionably the best technique for treating the arthrogrypotic congenital vertical tali. When comparing them to older patients who had undergone a single-stage open release/reduction, he has found that the latter are extremely stiff, with residual hind foot valgus and forefoot abductus. Even those Dobbs-treated feet that have developed a relapse continue to be flexible enough for repeat casting. In the past, the author had not paid enough attention to the subluxated calcaneocuboid joint, which led to many relapses. Now, during the casting phase, he closely evaluates the foot for concomitant calcaneocuboid subluxations, and in those cases, tries to persuade the cuboid to move in a more plantar direction as well. At surgery, the author will close, reduce, and pin the calcaneocuboid joint.

SUMMARY

Arthrogryposis and myelomeningocele foot deformities are challenging both to obtain and to maintain correction. The myelomeningocele clubfeet and congenital vertical tali are very similar to the arthrogrypotic ones, but their lack of protective sensation can complicate brace wear, particularly if the foot has lost all flexibility. Treatment strategies should center on methods that maintain flexibility.

Myelomeningocele foot deformities with an underlying dynamic component (equinus, calcaneus, calcaneovalgus) should be corrected early with serial casting and possibly limited tenotomies and maintained with constant bracing. Every attempt should be made to forestall larger procedures until the child is nearing maturity.

Relapse rates for arthrogrypotic and myelomeningocele clubfeet are high and should be expected regardless of the method of treatment. Although the natural preference is for a procedure that can be a once-and-done solution, at this time no such procedure is known. Because the clubfoot that relapses after cast correction can usually be corrected again by casting with little morbidity to the foot, the author considers this to be the best overall treatment strategy, until one is identified with relapse rates less than 5%.

REFERENCES

1. Swaroop VT, Dias L. Orthopedic management of spina bifida. Part I: hip, knee, and rotational deformities. J Child Orthop 2009;3(6):441–9.
2. Swaroop VT, Dias L. Orthopaedic management of spina bifida-part II: foot and ankle deformities. J Child Orthop 2011;5(6):403–14.
3. Parker SE, Mai CT, Canfield MA, et al. Updated National Birth Prevalence estimates for selected birth defects in the United States, 2004-2006. Birth Defects Res A Clin Mol Teratol 2010;88(12):1008–16.

4. Sharrard WJ, Zachary RB, Lorber J. Survival and paralysis in open myelomeningocele with special reference to the time of repair of the spinal lesion. Dev Med Child Neurol 1967;(Suppl 13):35–50.

5. Akbar M, Bresch B, Seyler TM, et al. Management of orthopaedic sequelae of congenital spinal disorders. J Bone Joint Surg Am 2009;91(Suppl 6):87–100.

6. Frischhut B, Stöckl B, Landauer F, et al. Foot deformities in adolescents and young adults with spina bifida. J Pediatr Orthop B 2000;9(3):161–9.

7. Thomson JD, Segal LS. Orthopedic management of spina bifida. Dev Disabil Res Rev 2010;16(1):96–103.

8. Broughton NS, Graham G, Menelaus MB. The high incidence of foot deformity in patients with high-level spina bifida. J Bone Joint Surg Br 1994;76(4): 548–50.

9. Frawley PA, Broughton NS, Menelaus MB. Incidence and type of hindfoot deformities in patients with low-level spina bifida. J Pediatr Orthop 1998;18(3):312–3.

10. Sharrard WJ. The orthopaedic surgery of spina bifida. Clin Orthop Relat Res 1973;(92):195–213.

11. Sharrard WJ, Grosfield I. The management of deformity and paralysis of the foot in myelomeningocele. J Bone Joint Surg Br 1968;50(3):456–65.

12. de Carvalho Neto J, Dias LS, Gabrieli AP. Congenital talipes equinovarus in spina bifida: treatment and results. J Pediatr Orthop 1996;16(6):782–5.

13. Flynn JM, Herrera-Soto JA, Ramirez NF, et al. Clubfoot release in myelodysplasia. J Pediatr Orthop B 2004;13(4):259–62.

14. Fraser RK, Hoffman EB. Calcaneus deformity in the ambulant patient with myelomeningocele. J Bone Joint Surg Br 1991;73(6):994–7.

15. Fucs PM, Svartman C, Santili C, et al. Results in the treatment of paralytic calcaneus-valgus feet with the Westin technique. Int Orthop 2007;31(4):555–60.

16. Malhotra D, Puri R, Owen R. Valgus deformity of the ankle in children with spina bifida aperta. J Bone Joint Surg Br 1984;66(3):381–5.

17. Torosian CM, Dias LS. Surgical treatment of severe hindfoot valgus by medial displacement osteotomy of the os calcis in children with myelomeningocele. J Pediatr Orthop 2000;20(2):226–9.

18. Abraham E, Lubicky JP, Songer MN, et al. Supramalleolar osteotomy for ankle valgus in myelomeningocele. J Pediatr Orthop 1996;16(6):774–81.

19. Burkus JK, Moore DW, Raycroft JF. Valgus deformity of the ankle in myelodysplastic patients. Correction by stapling of the medial part of the distal tibial physis. J Bone Joint Surg Am 1983;65(8):1157–62.

20. Westcott MA, Dynes MC, Remer EM, et al. Congenital and acquired orthopedic abnormalities in patients with myelomeningocele. Radiographics 1992;12(6): 1155–73.

21. Harris MB, Banta JV. Cost of skin care in the myelomeningocele population. J Pediatr Orthop 1990;10(3):355–61.

22. Maynard MJ, Weiner LS, Burke SW. Neuropathic foot ulceration in patients with myelodysplasia. J Pediatr Orthop 1992;12(6):786–8.

23. Roach JW, Short BF, Saltzman HM. Adult consequences of spina bifida: a cohort study. Clin Orthop Relat Res 2011;469(5):1246–52.

24. Chalayon O, Adams A, Dobbs MB. Minimally invasive approach for the treatment of non-isolated congenital vertical talus. J Bone Joint Surg Am 2012; 94(11):e73.

25. Gerlach DJ, Gurnett CA, Limpaphayom N, et al. Early results of the Ponseti method for the treatment of clubfoot associated with myelomeningocele. J Bone Joint Surg Am 2009;91(6):1350–9.

26. Bartonek A, Eriksson M, Gutierrez-Farewik EM. A new carbon fibre spring orthosis for children with plantarflexor weakness. Gait Posture 2007;25(4):652–6.
27. Vankoski SJ, Michaud S, Dias L. External tibial torsion and the effectiveness of the solid ankle-foot orthoses. J Pediatr Orthop 2000;20(3):349–55.
28. Wolf SI, Alimusaj M, Rettig O, et al. Dynamic assist by carbon fiber spring AFOs for patients with myelomeningocele. Gait Posture 2008;28(1):175–7.
29. Omeroglu S, Peker T, Omeroğlu H, et al. Intrauterine structure of foot muscles in talipes equinovarus due to high-level myelomeningocele: a light microscopic study in fetal cadavers. J Pediatr Orthop B 2004;13(4):263–7.
30. Dias LS, Stern LS. Talectomy in the treatment of resistant talipes equinovarus deformity in myelomeningocele and arthrogryposis. J Pediatr Orthop 1987; 7(1):39–41.
31. Janicki JA, Narayanan UG, Harvey B, et al. Treatment of neuromuscular and syndrome-associated (nonidiopathic) clubfeet using the Ponseti method. J Pediatr Orthop 2009;29(4):393–7.
32. Segev E, Ezra E, Yaniv M, et al. V osteotomy and Ilizarov technique for residual idiopathic or neurogenic clubfeet. J Orthop Surg (Hong Kong) 2008;16(2): 215–9.
33. Trumble T, Banta JV, Raycroft JF, et al. Talectomy for equinovarus deformity in myelodysplasia. J Bone Joint Surg Am 1985;67(1):21–9.
34. Crawford AH, Marxen JL, Osterfeld DL. The Cincinnati incision: a comprehensive approach for surgical procedures of the foot and ankle in childhood. J Bone Joint Surg Am 1982;64(9):1355–8.
35. Bassett GS, Mazur KU, Sloan GM. Soft-tissue expander failure in severe equinovarus foot deformity. J Pediatr Orthop 1993;13(6):744–8.
36. Menelaus MB. Talectomy for equinovarus deformity in arthrogryposis and spina bifida. J Bone Joint Surg Br 1971;53(3):468–73.
37. Segal LS, Mann DC, Feiwell E, et al. Equinovarus deformity in arthrogryposis and myelomeningocele: evaluation of primary talectomy. Foot Ankle Int 1989; 10(1):12–6.
38. Sherk HH, Ames MD. Talectomy in the treatment of the myelomeningocele patient. Clin Orthop Relat Res 1975;(110):218–22.
39. Sherk HH, Marchinski LJ, Clancy M, et al. Ground reaction forces on the plantar surface of the foot after talectomy in the myelomeningocele. J Pediatr Orthop 1989;9(3):269–75.
40. Cooper RR, Capello W. Talectomy. A long-term follow-up evaluation. Clin Orthop Relat Res 1985;(201):32–5.
41. Legaspi J, Li YH, Chow W, et al. Talectomy in patients with recurrent deformity in club foot. A long-term follow-up study. J Bone Joint Surg Br 2001;83(3):384–7.
42. van Bosse HJ. Treatment of the neglected and relapsed clubfoot. Clin Podiatr Med Surg 2013;30(4):513–30.
43. Correll J, Forth A. Correction of severe clubfoot by the Ilizarov method. Foot Ankle Surg 1996;2:27–32.
44. Grant AD, Atar D, Lehman WB. The Ilizarov technique in correction of complex foot deformities. Clin Orthop Relat Res 1992;(280):94–103.
45. Shingade VU, Shingade RV, Ughade SN. Single-stage correction for clubfoot associated with myelomeningocele in older children: early results. Curr Orthop Pract 2014;25(1):64–70.
46. Bensahela H, Kuo K, Duhaime M, et al. Outcome evaluation of the treatment of clubfoot: the international language of clubfoot. J Pediatr Orthop B 2003;12(4): 269–71.

47. Walker G. The early management of varus feet in myelomeningocele. J Bone Joint Surg Br 1971;53(3):462–7.
48. Dimeglio A, Canavese F. The French functional physical therapy method for the treatment of congenital clubfoot. J Pediatr Orthop B 2012;21(1):28–39.
49. Ponseti IV. Congenital clubfoot: fundamentals of treatment. New York: Oxford University Press Inc; 1996.
50. Ponseti IV, Smoley EN. Congenital club foot: the results of treatment. J Bone Joint Surg Am 1963;45(2):261–75, 344.
51. Gurnett CA, Boehm S, Connolly A, et al. Impact of congenital talipes equinovarus etiology on treatment outcomes. Dev Med Child Neurol 2008;50(7):498–502.
52. Moroney PJ, Noël J, Fogarty EE, et al. A single-center prospective evaluation of the Ponseti method in nonidlopathic congenital talipes equinovarus. J Pediatr Orthop 2012;32(6):636–40.
53. Franke J, Grill F, Hein G, et al. Correction of clubfoot relapse using Ilizarov's apparatus in children 8-15 years old. Arch Orthop Trauma Surg 1990;110(1):33–7.
54. Grill F, Franke J. The Ilizarov distractor for the correction of relapsed or neglected clubfoot. J Bone Joint Surg Br 1987;69(4):593–7.
55. Lamm BM, Standard SC, Galley IJ, et al. External fixation for the foot and ankle in children. Clin Podiatr Med Surg 2006;23(1):137–66, ix.
56. Tripathy SK, Saini R, Sudes P, et al. Application of the Ponseti principle for deformity correction in neglected and relapsed clubfoot using the Ilizarov fixator. J Pediatr Orthop B 2011;20(1):26–32.
57. Park KB, Park HW, Joo SY, et al. Surgical treatment of calcaneal deformity in a select group of patients with myelomeningocele. J Bone Joint Surg Am 2008; 90(10):2140 50.
58. Rodrigues RC, Dias LS. Calcaneus deformity in spina bifida: results of anterolateral release. J Pediatr Orthop 1992;12(4):461–4.
59. Galli M, Albertini G, Romei M, et al. Gait analysis in children affected by myelomeningocele: comparison of the various levels of lesion. Funct Neurol 2002; 17(4):203–10.
60. Bliss DG, Menelaus MB. The results of transfer of the tibialis anterior to the heel in patients who have a myelomeningocele. J Bone Joint Surg Am 1986;68(8): 1258–64.
61. Dias LS. Valgus deformity of the ankle joint: pathogenesis of fibular shortening. J Pediatr Orthop 1985;5(2):176–80.
62. Dias LS. Ankle valgus in children with myelomeningocele. Dev Med Child Neurol 1978;20(5):627–33.
63. Banta JV, Sutherland DH, Wyatt M. Anterior tibial transfer to the os calcis with Achilles tenodesis for calcaneal deformity in myelomeningocele. J Pediatr Orthop 1981;1(2):125–30.
64. Georgiadis GM, Aronson DD. Posterior transfer of the anterior tibial tendon in children who have a myelomeningocele. J Bone Joint Surg Am 1990;72(3): 392–8.
65. Turner JW, Cooper RR. Posterior transposition of tibialis anterior through the interosseous membrane. Clin Orthop Relat Res 1971;79:71–4.
66. Janda JP, Skinner SR, Barto PS. Posterior transfer of tibialis anterior in low-level myelodysplasia. Dev Med Child Neurol 1984;26(1):100–3.
67. Stott NS, Zionts LE, Gronley JK, et al. Tibialis anterior transfer for calcaneal deformity: a postoperative gait analysis. J Pediatr Orthop 1996;16(6):792–8.
68. Bradley GW, Coleman SS. Treatment of the calcaneocavus foot deformity. J Bone Joint Surg Am 1981;63(7):1159–66.

69. Wenz W, Bruckner T, Akbar M. Complete tendon transfer and inverse Lambrinudi arthrodesis: preliminary results of a new technique for the treatment of paralytic pes calcaneus. Foot Ankle Int 2008;29(7):683–9.

70. Badelon O, Bensahel H. Subtalar posterior displacement osteotomy of the calcaneus: a preliminary report of seven cases. J Pediatr Orthop 1990;10(3): 401–4.

71. Mitchell GP. Posterior displacement osteotomy of the calcaneus. J Bone Joint Surg Br 1977;59(2):233–5.

72. Koutsogiannis E. Treatment of mobile flat foot by displacement osteotomy of the calcaneus. J Bone Joint Surg Br 1971;53(1):96–100.

73. Levitt RL, Canale ST, Gartland JJ. Surgical correction of foot deformity in the older patient with myelomeningocele. Orthop Clin North Am 1974;5(1):19–29.

74. Gallien R, Morin F, Marquis F. Subtalar arthrodesis in children. J Pediatr Orthop 1989;9(1):59–63.

75. Aronson DD, Middleton DL. Extra-articular subtalar arthrodesis with cancellous bone graft and internal fixation for children with myelomeningocele. Dev Med Child Neurol 1991;33(3):232–40.

76. Arkin AM, Katz JF. The effects of pressure on epiphyseal growth; the mechanism of plasticity of growing bone. J Bone Joint Surg Am 1956;38-A(5):1056–76.

77. Westin GW. Tendon transfers about the foot, ankle, and hip in the paralyzed lower extremity. J Bone Joint Surg Am 1965;47(7):1430–43.

78. Westin GW, Dingeman RD, Gausewitz SH. The results of tenodesis of the tendo achillis to the fibula for paralytic pes calcaneus. J Bone Joint Surg Am 1988; 70(3):320–8.

79. Stevens PM, Toomey E. Fibular-Achilles tenodesis for paralytic ankle valgus. J Pediatr Orthop 1988;8(2):169–75.

80. Stevens PM, Belle RM. Screw epiphysiodesis for ankle valgus. J Pediatr Orthop 1997;17(1):9–12.

81. Sharrard WJ, Webb J. Supra-malleolar wedge osteotomy of the tibia in children with myelomeningocele. J Bone Joint Surg Br 1974;56B(3):458–61.

82. Lubicky JP, Altiok H. Transphyseal osteotomy of the distal tibia for correction of valgus/varus deformities of the ankle. J Pediatr Orthop 2001;21(1):80–8.

83. Drennan JC, Sharrard WJ. The pathological anatomy of convex pes valgus. J Bone Joint Surg Br 1971;53(3):455–61.

84. Kodros SA, Dias LS. Single-stage surgical correction of congenital vertical talus. J Pediatr Orthop 1999;19(1):42–8.

85. Ogata K, Schoenecker PL, Sheridan J. Congenital vertical talus and its familial occurrence: an analysis of 36 patients. Clin Orthop Relat Res 1979;(139): 128–32.

86. Dobbs MB, Purcell DB, Nunley R, et al. Early results of a new method of treatment for idiopathic congenital vertical talus. J Bone Joint Surg Am 2006;88(6): 1192–200.

87. Dobbs MB, Purcell DB, Nunley R, et al. Early results of a new method of treatment for idiopathic congenital vertical talus. Surgical technique. J Bone Joint Surg Am 2007;89(Suppl 2 Pt.1):111–21.

88. Hall JG. Arthrogryposis multiplex congenita: etiology, genetics, classification, diagnostic approach, and general aspects. J Pediatr Orthop B 1997;6(3): 159–66.

89. Bevan WP, Hall JG, Bamshad M, et al. Arthrogryposis multiplex congenita (amyoplasia): an orthopaedic perspective. J Pediatr Orthop 2007;27(5): 594–600.

90. Carlson WO, Speck GJ, Vicari V, et al. Arthrogryposis multiplex congenita. A long-term follow-up study. Clin Orthop Relat Res 1985;(194):115–23.
91. Drummond DS, Cruess RL. The management of the foot and ankle in arthrogryposis multiplex congenita. J Bone Joint Surg Br 1978;60(1):96–9.
92. Hall JG, Reed SD, Driscoll EP. Part I. Amyoplasia: a common, sporadic condition with congenital contractures. Am J Med Genet 1983;15(4):571–90.
93. Zimbler S, Craig CL. The arthrogrypotic foot plan of management and results of treatment. Foot Ankle 1983;3(4):211–9.
94. Guidera KJ, Drennan JC. Foot and ankle deformities in arthrogryposis multiplex congenita. Clin Orthop Relat Res 1985;(194):93–8.
95. Hahn G. Arthrogryposis. Pediatric review and habilitative aspects. Clin Orthop Relat Res 1985;(194):104–14.
96. Khan MA, Chinoy MA. Treatment of severe and neglected clubfoot with a double zigzag incision: outcome of 21 feet in 15 patients followed up between 1 and 5 years. J Foot Ankle Surg 2006;45(3):177–81.
97. Niki H, Staheli LT, Mosca VS. Management of clubfoot deformity in amyoplasia. J Pediatr Orthop 1997;17(6):803–7.
98. Palmer PM, MacEwen GD, Bowen JR, et al. Passive motion therapy for infants with arthrogryposis. Clin Orthop Relat Res 1985;(194):54–9.
99. Sells JM, Jaffe KM, Hall JG. Amyoplasia, the most common type of arthrogryposis: the potential for good outcome. Pediatrics 1996;97(2):225–31.
100. Simons GW. Complete subtalar release in club feet. Part I–a preliminary report. J Bone Joint Surg Am 1985;67(7):1044–55.
101. Södergård J, Ryöppy S. Foot deformities in arthrogryposis multiplex congenita. J Pediatr Orthop 1994;14(6):768–72.
102. Widmann RF, Do TT, Burke SW. Radical soft-tissue release of the arthrogrypotic clubfoot. J Pediatr Orthop B 2005;14(2):111–5.
103. Williams P. The management of arthrogryposis. Orthop Clin North Am 1978;9(1):67–88.
104. Cassis N, Capdevila R. Talectomy for clubfoot in arthrogryposis. J Pediatr Orthop 2000;20(5):652–5.
105. D'Souza H, Aroojis A, Yagnik MG. Rotation fasciocutaneous flap for neglected clubfoot: a new technique. J Pediatr Orthop 1998;18(3):319–22.
106. Hsu LC, Jaffray D, Leong JC. Talectomy for club foot in arthrogryposis. J Bone Joint Surg Br 1984;66(5):694–6.
107. Green AD, Fixsen JA, Lloyd-Roberts GC. Talectomy for arthrogryposis multiplex congenita. J Bone Joint Surg Br 1984;66(5):697–9.
108. Solund K, Sonne-Holm S, Kjolbye JE. Talectomy for equinovarus deformity in arthrogryposis. A 13 (2-20) year review of 17 feet. Acta Orthop Scand 1991;62(4):372–4.
109. Nicomedez FP, Li YH, Leong JC. Tibiocalcaneal fusion after talectomy in arthrogrypotic patients. J Pediatr Orthop 2003;23(5):654–7.
110. D'Souza H, Aroojis A, Chawara GS. Talectomy in arthrogryposis: analysis of results. J Pediatr Orthop 1998;18(6):760–4.
111. El Barbary H, Abdel Ghani H, Hegazy M. Correction of relapsed or neglected clubfoot using a simple Ilizarov frame. Int Orthop 2004;28(3):183–6.
112. Brunner R, Hefti F, Tgetgel JD. Arthrogrypotic joint contracture at the knee and the foot: correction with a circular frame. J Pediatr Orthop B 1997;6(3):192–7.
113. Choi IH, Yang MS, Chung CY, et al. The treatment of recurrent arthrogrypotic club foot in children by the Ilizarov method. A preliminary report. J Bone Joint Surg Br 2001;83(5):731–7.

114. Morcuende JA, Dobbs MB, Frick SL. Results of the Ponseti method in patients with clubfoot associated with arthrogryposis. Iowa Orthop J 2008;28:22–6.
115. van Bosse HJ, Marangoz S, Lehman WB, et al. Correction of arthrogrypotic clubfoot with a modified Ponseti technique. Clin Orthop Relat Res 2009; 467(5):1283–93.
116. Boehm S, Limpaphayom N, Alaee F, et al. Early results of the Ponseti method for the treatment of clubfoot in distal arthrogryposis. J Bone Joint Surg Am 2008; 90(7):1501–7.
117. Ponseti IV, Zhivkov M, Davis N, et al. Treatment of the complex idiopathic clubfoot. Clin Orthop Relat Res 2006;451:171–6.
118. Aroojis AJ, King MM, Donohoe M, et al. Congenital vertical talus in arthrogryposis and other contractural syndromes. Clin Orthop Relat Res 2005;(434):26–32.
119. Ramanoudjame M, Loriaut P, Seringe R, et al. The surgical treatment of children with congenital convex foot (vertical talus): evaluation of midtarsal surgical release and open reduction. Bone Joint J 2014;96-B(6):837–44.
120. Wright J, Coggings D, Maizen C, et al. Reverse Ponseti-type treatment for children with congenital vertical talus: comparison between idiopathic and teratological patients. Bone Joint J 2014;96-B(2):274–8.

Cavus Foot

Monica Paschoal Nogueira, PhD, MD[a],*, Fernando Farcetta, MD[b],
Alexandre Zuccon, MD[b]

KEYWORDS

- Foot deformities • Cavus foot • Charcot–Marie–Tooth • Foot osteotomies

KEY POINTS

- Presentation of cavus foot requires complete physical examination and imaging to look for neurologic abnormalities.
- Charcot–Marie–Tooth disease presents in the young patient with symptoms such as abnormal gait, forefoot pain, and ankle instability.
- It is important to describe whether a cavus foot is flexible or rigid to decide on the indication for soft tissue surgery such as tendon transfers, usually associated with bony procedures.
- In cavus foot evaluation, it is important to determine the apex of the deformity (or deformities) to choose the best operative technique.
- Joint-sparing surgery such as tarsectomies are preferable alternative to triple arthrodesis.

INTRODUCTION

Cavus is the foot deformity described as a high plantar arch and a fixed forefoot equinus. Pronation of the first ray can also occur, and calcaneous could be in varus—cavovarus (most common)—or calcaneus–calcaneocavus. The heel could also be less commonly in valgus and/or equinus. Neurologic evaluation is mandatory, because cavus deformity is often associated with different neurologic entities, responsible for the imbalance of synergistic intrinsic and extrinsic muscles. Cavus deformity could be progressive or caused by paralytic soft tissue diseases, osteoarticular diseases, or trauma (**Figs. 1–3, Table 1**).

MORPHOLOGY

Polymorphism is the rule owing to the diversity of etiologic factors.

The authors have nothing to disclose.
[a] Pediatric Orthopaedics, Department of Orthopaedic, HSPE State Public Hospital, 1755 Borges Lagoa St., Vila Clementino, São Paulo 04038-034, Brazil; [b] Department of Orthopaedic, AACD – Association for Care of Disabled Child, 724 Professor Ascendino Reis Avenue, Ibirapuera, São Paulo 04027-000, Brazil
* Corresponding author.
E-mail address: monipn@uol.com.br

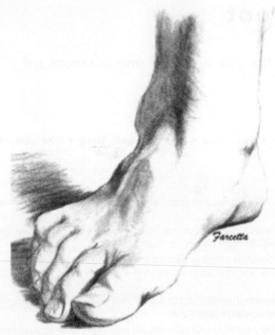

Fig. 1. Cavus foot.

Sagittal Plane Deformities

- *Posterior cavus foot* (calcaneus or vertical calcaneus deformity) is very disabling, and is caused by weakness of the Achilles tendon.
- *Anterior cavus foot* is the most common deformity. The metatarsals are in plantar flexion, specially the first ray, associated with claw toes. The intrinsic muscles are often weak and there is retraction of plantar soft tissue.

Claw toes are explained by disturbance of the foot muscular balance. Normally, intrinsic muscles flex the metatarsophalangeal joints and extend the interphalangeal joints. When the long flexor is activated over an extended toe, it glides over the metatarsal head and prevents forefoot flexion on the hindfoot.

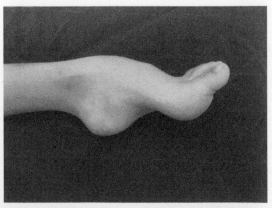

Fig. 2. Clinical aspect of a cavus foot in Charcot–Marie–Tooth disease.

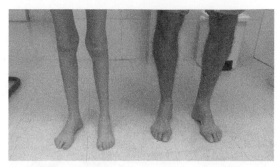

Fig. 3. Charcot–Marie–Tooth disease (type 1) is autosomal dominant; father and son present with cavus foot.

Absence of lumbrical muscles causes long flexors to act with no support of metatarsal heads, and that results in extension of metatarsophalangeal joints and hyperflexion of interphalangeal joints[1] (**Fig. 4**).

Extrinsic muscle imbalance
- Weak anterior tibialis tendon.
- Strong peroneus longus.
- Strong extensor hallucis longus (windlass mechanism).
- Weak triceps surae may result in the long toe flexors trying to compensate during stance phase, worsening the forefoot equinus.
- Strong tibialis posterior overcomes eversion strength (weak peroneus brevis) and results in varus of the calcaneus.

Coronal Plane Deformities

Calcaneus is commonly in varus and, together with the equinus forefoot, is part of the tripod that is typical of cavus foot.

Table 1
Cavus foot etiology

Neurologic	Osteoarticular Changes	Soft Tissue Contractures
Charcot–Marie–Tooth disease	Congenital cavus foot	Ledderhose disease
Polyneuritic syndromes	Rheumatoid arthritis	Scar tissue, iatrogenic
Dejerine–Sottas disease	Trauma	Burns
Friedrich ataxia	Inadequate use of shoes	Vascular lesions
Roussy–Levy syndrome	—	—
Stumpell–Lorrain disease	—	—
Pierre–Marie heredotaxy	—	—
Cerebral palsy	—	—
Parkinson disease	—	—
Poliomyelitis	—	—
Myelomeningocele	—	—
Nerve trauma	—	—
Tumors	—	—
Leprosy	—	—
Hysterical cavus	—	—

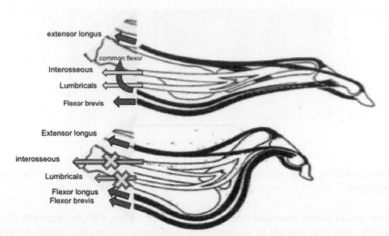

Fig. 4. Muscle forces in the normal foot and muscle forces in the abnormal foot, with weak intrinsic muscles. (*From* González Casanova JC. Pie cavo. En Viladot A, editor. Diez lecciones sobre patología del pie. Barcelona (Spain): Masson S.A; 1979. p. 95; with permission.)

CLINICAL PRESENTATION

Cavus deformity is usually insidious and happens before puberty. It could be unilateral or bilateral, and gait disturbance could be among the initial findings. Swing phase shows a deformed foot, heel strike does not happen, and the forefoot touches the ground before the hindfoot. Shoes present wear in the anterior part of the sole and the dorsal aspect is usually deformed; walking can be unstable, and falls are frequent.

Initially, cavus foot can be flexible, and becomes more rigid over time with soft tissues contractures. Pain occurs as the weight bearing is divided into the tripod surface (less area of weigh bearing, more pressure per unit of area), excessive pressure causes hygroma and calluses, and can be complicated by sesamoiditis.

- Detailed neurologic examination
  - Attention to the spine (deformities or midline defect, dimple, or hairy patch)
- Mobility of hindfoot and forefoot
- Muscle testing to detect imbalance is important to correct to avoid relapses **(Fig. 5)**
- Coleman bloc test 1977[2]
  - Assesses flexibility of hindfoot varus when forefoot is rigid.
  - If the forefoot is placed off the bloc, and calcaneous moves from varus to valgus, subtalar joint is flexible and only forefoot surgery is indicated; if calcaneous do not move into valgus, hindfoot deformity is also rigid and must be addressed as well **(Fig. 6)**
- Kelikian's test
  - Tension of plantar fascia can be obtained with passive hyperextension of metatarsophalangeal joint, and if deformity is not rigid, claw toes correct

COMPLEMENTARY EXAMINATIONS
Gait Analysis

Visual analysis and gait laboratory are useful. Alterations in swing and stance phases should be analyzed.

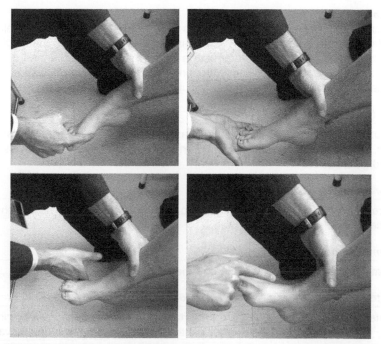

Fig. 5. Clinical examination for motor strength and activity is very important to detect imbalance that must be addressed to prevent relapse.

Radiographic Evaluation

Anteroposterlor and lateral films of the spine are important to investigate a neurologic etiology.

Normal anatomy of the foot

In the sagittal plane, the angle between the longitudinal axis of calcaneus and forefoot is 130° (Hibb's angle); the apex of this angle is close to Chopart joint. The angle between the horizontal plane and metatarsal or forefoot axis is 22°. The hindfoot angle between the horizontal plane and the axis of the heel is 28° (calcaneal pitch). The angle between the talar axis and horizontal plane is 24°. Talus and first metatarsal are aligned (Méary's line).

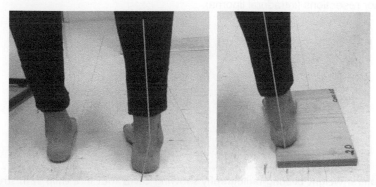

Fig. 6. Coleman bloc test in flexible cavovarus foot.

In the cavus foot

The calcaneal pitch is increased in the cavus foot, as well as the angle determined by the metatarsal and horizontal plane (metatarsals are more flexed). The longitudinal axis of calcaneus and forefoot determine a lower magnitude angle, and in consequence a shorter foot. Méary's line is broken, and this angle determines the apex of cavus deformity (center of rotation and angulation)[3] (**Fig. 7**).

Podometry

Podometry is the reading of the pressure areas of the foot. It is performed in a standing position. The clinical inspection of plantar surface can outline points with excess pressure and glabrous skin.

Podobarometry

Pressure points can be analyzed during gait or stance phase, and are usually shown in color scale.

Electromyography

Electromyography is helpful to unfold peripheric nerve function compromise.

Computed Tomography and MRI for Neurologic Evaluation

Computed tomography and MRI are important for the investigation of progressive causes, including intramedular lipoma, central nervous system tumors, or vascular lesions.

CONSERVATIVE TREATMENT

- Physical therapy: to keep feet flexible and for gait reeducation.
- Casting in progressive abduction: used in previously operated feet; can be efficient to treat nonprogressive deformities.[4]
- Insoles: total contact principle; minimize hyperpressure points, callosities, and pain; also used in retrometatarsal bar and pronation wedge.
- Customized shoes: wide with a high forefoot.

SURGICAL TREATMENT
Neurosurgical

Use an approach to reduce spasticity (intratecal baclofen, selective dorsal rhizotomy), and tumor resections (intradural lipoma).

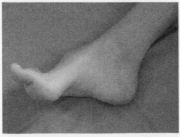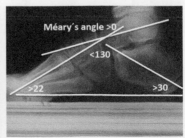

Fig. 7. Lateral weight bearing radiography showing cavus foot in a child with structured cavus deformity.

Orthopedic Treatment

The 2 main goals are correction of the deformity and strength balance. Several procedures can be used for correction of the deformity, depending on flexibility and of the foot location of deformity apex, presence or absence of sensibility, and severity of deformity. They must be combined in a customized way to treat each foot.[5–7]

SOFT TISSUE PROCEDURES
Steindler Plantar Release for Mild and Flexible Cases

A medial plantar incision is made on skin and fat tissue; the plantar fascia is cut horizontally from medial to lateral. Intrinsic plantar muscles (abductor hallucis, flexor digitorum brevis, quadratus plantae, and abductor minimi digitorum) are detached from calcaneus and plantar ligaments are released as well as most of the plantar longus ligament (**Fig. 8**).

Fasciectomy

Fasciectomy accomplishes a complete resection of the plantar fascia, through a longitudinal plantar incision.

Tendon Transfers

The aim is to balance the forces on the foot; importantly, the foot must be flexible and the tendon transferred must be strong.

Jones Procedure

The Jones procedure includes transfer of the long extensor hallucis to the neck of the first metatarsal, elevating the first ray. It is usually accompanied by interphalangeal joint fusion (**Fig. 9**).[8]

Claw Toes Treatment

When claw toes are flexible, flexor tenotomies could be indicated to treat distal deformities. If the metatarsal is plantar flexed, the Jones procedure can elevate the metatarsal head. If claw toes are rigid, bony procedures such as fusions can correct the deformity.

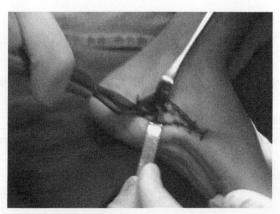

Fig. 8. Steindler medial plantar release.

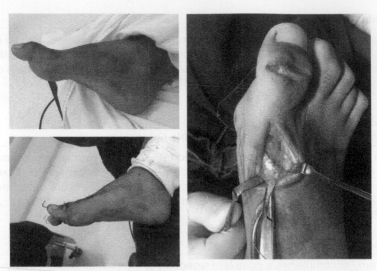

Fig. 9. Jones procedure. Correction of flexible cavus foot by transfer of the long extensor hallucis to the neck of the first metatarsal.

FOOT OSTEOTOMIES

Decision making is based on the rigidity of foot and location of the apex of deformity (calculated with a lateral weight-bearing radiograph). The apex can be found in the intersection of talar and first metatarsal lines.

First Metatarsal Extension Osteotomy

First metatarsal extension osteotomy is often indicated owing to flexed first ray. Attention must be paid to the proximal physis in skeletally immature patients. In children, it is often fixed with Kirschner wires.

Medial Cuneiform Osteotomy

Dorsal closing wedge or plantar open wedge osteotomy may be performed when the metatarsal physis is open or when the apex of deformity is at the level of medial cuneiform.

Calcaneus Osteotomies

- *Dwyer:* lateral wedge resection of calcaneus is a good indication to treat varus of hindfoot.
- *Samilson:* crescentic osteotomy for treatment of calcaneus deformity (vertical calcaneous; **Fig. 10**).[9]

Tarsectomies or Midfoot Osteotomies

These procedures are indicated in rigid, multiple operated and severe feet, usually in adolescents; they follow the same principles of adult cavus feet.

- *Japas:* V osteotomy of tarsus, with a dorsal incision.[10]
- *Mubarak:* salvage procedure with naviculectomy and dorsal wedge resection of cuboid.[11]
- *Talectomy:* often used in rigid arthrogrypotic feet and difficult clubfeet.

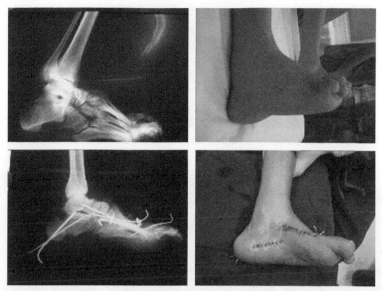

Fig. 10. Samilson osteotomy for calcaneocavus foot. Cole osteotomy of middle foot is also shown.

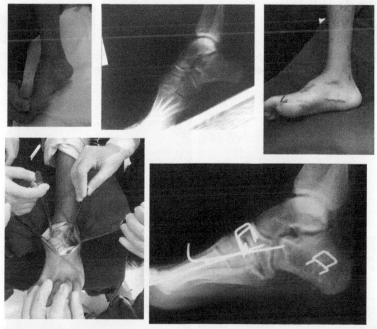

Fig. 11. Cole osteotomy (incision between the extensor digitorum longus and long hallucis extensor), Dwyer calcaneous osteotomy, and plantar and posteromedial release for correction of a cavus foot.

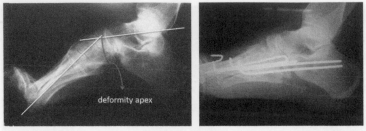

Fig. 12. Cole osteotomy (anterior wedge resection) at the apex of deformity in the sagittal plane.

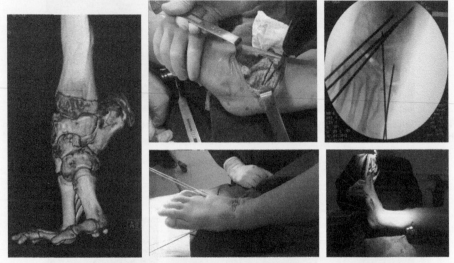

Fig. 13. Structured multioperated cavovarus foot (sequela of clubfoot treatment) corrected with partial talectomy, and another more distal wedge resection in the midfoot (Cole procedure).

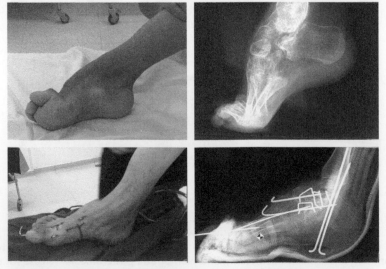

Fig. 14. Cavus foot in Charcot–Marie–Tooth disease treated by triple arthrodesis.

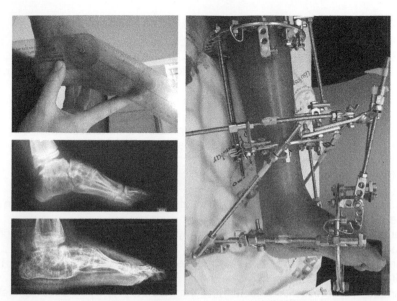

Fig. 15 Circular external fixation with V osteotomy to treat a multioperated rigid cavus foot in a 10-year-old girl. (Clinical preoperative aspect, preoperative and postoperative films, and aspect during treatment).

- *Akron:* midtarsal dome osteotomy; with a curved wedge, correction of deformity in the sagittal and frontal planes is possible.[12]
- *Cole:* anterior tarsal wedge osteotomy (**Figs. 11–13**).
- *Lelievre:* dorsal wedge including navicular and first cuneiform (with fusion) on the medial side, and another dorsal wedge of the cuboid (intraosseous).
- *Triple arthrodesis:* salvage procedure used more often in adolescents for deformities proximal to the midfoot[13] (**Fig. 14**).
- *Lambrinudi:* type of triple arthrodesis with resection of neck and head of talus, and plantar aspect of navicular.[14]

EXTERNAL FIXATION CORRECTION

With or without foot osteotomies, external fixation correction is based on Ilizarov principle of soft tissue distraction and distraction osteogenesis with gradual correction. It has the advantage of achieve correction of severe deformity of the foot (**Fig. 15**).[15] Currently, 6-axis external fixators have been used owing to versatility and modularity of frames, allowing for correction of complex deformities.

SUMMARY

Cavus foot is usually related to neurologic abnormalities and then requires complete clinical and imaging evaluation. It is important to identify whether the deformity is flexible or rigid, and combine different soft tissue and bony techniques to accomplish the best lasting results. On rigid feet, it is crucial to determine the apex of the deformity to guide the bony procedures indicated for each specific case. Tarsectomies are preferred to arthrodesis in these rigid feet with the aim of achieve a plantigrade foot.

REFERENCES

1. Myerson MS, Shereff MJ. The pathological anatomy claw and hammer toes. J Bone Joint Surg Am 1989;71(1):45–9.
2. Coleman SS, Chesnut WJ. A simple test for hindfoot flexibility in the cavovarus foot. Clin Orthop 1977;123:60–2.
3. Paley D. Principles of deformity correction. Berlin, Germany: Springer-Verlag, Heidelberg; 2002.
4. Nogueira MP, Ey Batlle AM, Alves CG. Is it possible to treat recurrent clubfoot with the Ponseti technique after posteromedial release?: a preliminary study. Clin Orthop Relat Res 2009;467(5):1298–305.
5. Schwend RM, Drenman JC. Cavus foot in children. J Am Acad Orthop Surg 2003; 11(3):201–11.
6. Mubarak SJ, Van Valin SE. Osteotomies of the foot for cavus deformities in children. J Pediatr Orthop 2009;29(3):294–9.
7. Parekh SG, editor. Foot and ankle surgery. New Delhi (India): Jaypee Brothers Medical Publishers; 2012.
8. Jones R. An operation for paralytic calcaneo-cavus. J Bone Joint Surg Am 1908; 25(4):(s2–5):371–6.
9. Samilson RL. Crescentic osteotomy of the os calcis for calcaneocavus feet. In: Bateman JE, editor. Foot science. Philadelphia: WB Saunders; 1976. p. 18–25.
10. Japas LM. Surgical treatment of pes cavus by V-osteotomy: preliminary report. J Bone Joint Surg Am 1968;50(5):927–44.
11. Mubarak SJ, Dimeglio A. Navicular excision and cuboid closing wedge for severe cavovarus foot deformities: a salvage procedure. J Pediatr Orthop 2011;31(5): 551–6.
12. Weiner DS, Morscher M, Junko JT, et al. The Akron dome midfoot osteotomy as a salvage procedure for the treatment of rigid pes cavus. J Pediatr Orthop 2008; 28(1):68–80.
13. Penny JN. The neglected clubfoot. Tech Orthop 2005;20(2):153–66.
14. Lambrinudi C. New operation on drop-foot. Br J Surg 1927;15:197–200.
15. Kirienko A, Villa A, Calhoun JH. Ilizarov technique for complex foot and ankle deformities. New York: Marcel Decker, Inc; 2004.

Neuromuscular Foot
Spastic Cerebral Palsy

 CrossMark

Mara S. Karamitopoulos, MD*, Lana Nirenstein, MD

KEYWORDS

- Cerebral palsy • Pes planovalgus • Equinovarus foot • Subtalar fusion
- Calcaneal lengthening

KEY POINTS

- Fixed equinus contracture owing to equal gastrocnemius and soleus contracture can be treated with open tendoachilles lengthening.
- Ankle valgus is a secondary deformity, but can be treated with medial epiphysiodesis if there is more than 10° of valgus and the child has sufficient growth remaining.
- Pes planovalgus is the most common foot deformity in diplegics and quadriplegics; surgical treatment includes lateral calcaneal lengthening and subtalar fusion in severe cases.
- Most equinovarus deformities improve with age, but can be treated with tendon transfers in older children if the foot passively corrects without residual fixed heel varus.
- Preoperative gait analysis can help to define the need for adjunctive tendon transfers or additional procedures proximal to the ankle.

Foot and ankle deformities are common in patients with cerebral palsy. Deformity can vary with degree of spasticity and anatomic classification (ie, diplegic vs quadriplegic). Ambulatory children will have problems that inhibit gait efficiency. Nonambulatory children typically have foot and ankle problems that can prevent comfortable shoe and orthotic wear.[1] Although hemiplegia more often leads to an equinovarus deformity, equinovalgus deformity is seen more commonly in children with spastic diplegia and quadriplegia.[2]

Equinus contracture occurs in children with spasticity owing to overpull of the dorsiflexors relative to ankle plantarflexors.[3] Articulating ankle–foot orthoses can be used in children with mild, flexible ankle equinus. In children where the equinus becomes fixed, botulinum toxin injections can be used to prevent or delay surgery. Children with fixed contracture who cannot dorsiflex to neutral despite bracing and botulinum toxin injections are considered candidates for operative intervention.

The authors have nothing to disclose.
Department of Orthopaedic Surgery, Maimonides Medical Center, Maimonides Bone & Joint Center, 6010 Bay Parkway, 7th Floor, Brooklyn, NY 11204, USA
* Corresponding author. Maimonides Bone & Joint Center, 6010 Bay Parkway, 7th Floor, Brooklyn, NY 11204.
E-mail address: mkaramit@gmail.com

Ankle valgus is typically a secondary deformity. The amount of ankle valgus is determined by measuring the tibiotalar angle on a weight-bearing anteroposterior view of the ankle. Radiographic features identified with ankle valgus include narrow distal fibular physis and a shortened fibula. Ankle valgus is effectively treated with epiphysiodesis of the medial malleolus. Guided growth is an effective option when the physis are open and the child has more than 2 years of growth remaining.

In planovalgus deformity, the hindfoot is in valgus with midfoot pronation and forefoot eversion. This segmental malalignment can decrease substantially the lever arm for the third rocker[4] and allows for less push-off power. Fusion procedures should be avoided if possible in children who are functional ambulators. Lateral column lengthening, either via lengthening at the calcaneal neck or performing an opening wedge osteotomy through the calcaneocuboid joint, should be used to correct the deformity. In children who have lesser functional demands with severe deformity, subtalar fusion can be added to lateral column lengthening with good results.[5] Intraoperative examination after subtalar fusion and calcaneal lengthening is critical to ensure that the normal balance of the foot is restored.

Spastic equinovarus deformity is caused by spasticity of the gastrocsoleus, posterior tibialis, and/or anterior tibialis. Nonoperative treatment is preferred in young children because mild varus can often progress to planovalgus as children grow into middle childhood and adolescence.[6] Varus deformity is more likely to progress in hemiplegics. Both the anterior tibialis and the posterior tibialis can drive the deformity. Before surgical intervention is undertaken, gait analysis with electromyographic (EMG) monitoring and pedobarographs can be helpful to determine which tendon is most overactive and out of phase. The treatment of a severely fixed varus deformity is triple arthrodesis.

OPERATIVE TECHNIQUES
Open Tendoachilles Lengthening

Several techniques exist to treat equinus contracture. Open tendoachilles lengthening should be performed in children with fixed equinus contracture in whom the gastrocnemius and soleus are equally contracted.

Preoperative planning
Preoperative physical examination determines extent of contracture in each muscle. Children with large differences in contracture between the gastrocnemius and the soleus are better treated with fractional gastrocnemius lengthening. Radiographs aid in confirming that there is no midfoot or forefoot involvement.

Patient positioning
Patients should be positioned supine with a tourniquet placed on the upper thigh. The tourniquet can be placed sterilely during the procedure if more proximal procedures are also planned.

Surgical approach and procedure
1. An incision is made along the medial aspect of the Achilles tendon. Straight posterior incisions should be avoided to prevent shoe and brace wear discomfort.
2. The fascia of the Achilles tendon is incised, and a retractor is placed around the tendon. The tendon is freed up from other soft tissue attachments.
3. The Achilles tendon is incised through its center (**Fig. 1**A). Care should be taken to ensure sufficient overlap after lengthening and allow for appropriate tension of the tendon (usually 3–4 cm central limb is needed).

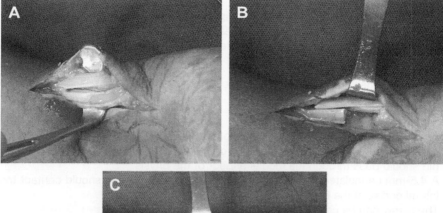

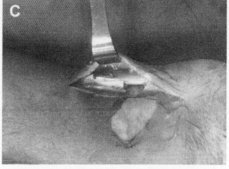

Fig. 1. Open tendoachilles Z-lengthening. (A) The Achilles tendon is incised through its center. (B) Z-lengthening allows the tendon to slide. (C) The tendon is sutured with moderate tension with foot in -10° dorsiflexion.

4. The distal segment of the tendon should be taken off laterally if the patient's hindfoot is in valgus and medially if the foot tends toward varus. The proximal segment is incised to the opposite side of the distal cut.
5. Gentle dorsiflexion of the foot allows tendon ends to slide (**Fig. 1**B). If the tendon does not slide as expected, the tendon ends may still be tethered to surrounding soft tissue.
6. The tendon should be repaired with absorbable suture while holding the foot in -10° of dorsiflexion (**Fig. 1**C). Forceps can be used to hold moderate tension on the ends of the tendon during repair.

Immediate postoperative care
The patient is immobilized in a weight-bearing short leg cast with the foot in neutral dorsiflexion for 6 weeks.

Rehabilitation and recovery
After cast removal, patients are allowed to bear weight as tolerated. A follow-up examination at 4 weeks after cast removal can reveal whether orthotics are still needed.

Ankle Epiphysiodesis Screw

Epiphysiodesis of the medial tibial physis is an effective tool to correct ankle valgus in patients with more than 2 years of growth remaining. A single cannulated screw in the medial malleolus can be inserted for epiphysiodesis. These children should be followed every few months with radiographs to determine timing of screw removal (when neutral alignment to slight overcorrection is restored).

Preoperative planning
Weight-bearing radiographs of the ankle can help to assess deformity. The tibiotalar axis should be measured. Children with greater than 10° of valgus who still have substantial growth potential are ideal candidates for this procedure.

Patient positioning
The patient is positioned supine on a radiolucent table. A tourniquet can be applied to be used if needed.

Surgical approach and procedure
1. A stab incision is made over the area of planned screw entry. A guidewire is inserted under fluoroscopic guidance through the tip of the medial malleolus. The pin should pass through the medial aspect of the physis.
2. A 4.5-mm cannulated screw is placed over the guidewire and should contact the lateral cortex of the tibia.
3. The screw can be countersunk to make it less prominent.

Immediate postoperative care
No postoperative immobilization is required.

Rehabilitation and recovery
No specific rehabilitation protocol is required. They should avoid wearing any braces while the incision is healing to prevent wound irritation or dehiscence.[7,8] Patient should be evaluated with radiographs every 4 to 6 months to evaluate correction. Most children require screw removal at some point.

Lateral Column Lengthening

Lengthening of the lateral column can be achieved by different methods, with the primary goal of correcting the hypermobility of the talus in the acetabulum pedis. Lengthening through calcaneal osteotomy is discussed here. The advantage of this osteotomy is that it preserves motion at the subtalar joint, which is helpful in patients with less severe deformity. It is not indicated as an isolated procedure in nonambulatory quadriplegics with severe deformity.

Preoperative planning
The child's Gross Motor Function Classification System level and ambulation potential should be evaluated carefully. Preoperative radiographs are helpful to evaluate bony deformity and degenerative changes. As mentioned, children who are nonambulatory are not ideal candidate for this procedure.

Patient positioning
The patient should be supine with a tourniquet placed proximally. A small bump can be added under the hip if patient's position makes access to the lateral foot difficult. If the use of iliac crest autograft is planned, this site should also be prepped out prior to the start of the procedure.

Surgical approach and procedure
1. Skin incision begins just proximal to the anterior border of the lateral malleolus and curved distally to the anterior border of peroneus brevis.
2. Subperiosteal dissection is carried out just anterior to peroneus brevis. The sinus tarsi is exposed and cleaned out (**Fig. 2A**). The area anterior to the middle facet is identified.
3. Dissection is carried out from the middle of the calcaneal tuberosity to the capsule of the calcaneocuboid joint. Do not violate the calcaneocuboid joint. The inferior

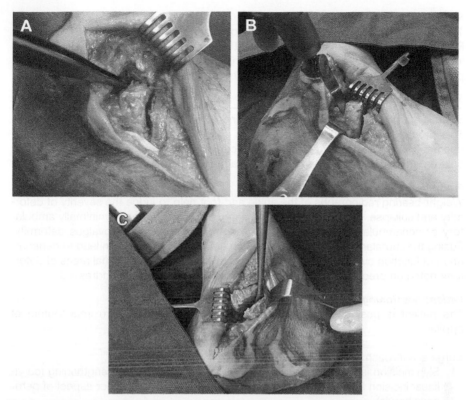

Fig. 2. Lateral calcaneal lengthening. (*A*) Forceps in the sinus tarsi that has been exposed and cleaned out. (*B*) Osteotomy is started just anterior to middle facet. In this specimen, the calcaneocuboid joint is to the right. (*C*) Osteotomy can be opened with a laminar spreader. Cobb elevator is within osteotomy site that has been opened.

aspect of the calcaneus should also be dissected out. Inferior soft tissues should be protected.
4. The osteotomy is started just anterior to the middle facet of the calcaneus in the transverse plane (perpendicular to the calcaneocuboid joint) with an oscillating saw (**Fig. 2**B). Once the osteotomy has been started, the medial cortex can be transected with an osteotome. Care should be taken to transect the calcaneus completely.
5. A lamina spreader or a Cobb elevator can be used to open the osteotomy site (**Fig. 2**C). The osteotomy should be opened until optimal correction has been obtained (corrected supination with forefoot adduction). Be careful not to overcorrect the deformity.
6. The site is now prepared for bone grafting. If use of autograft is planned, a tricortical iliac crest graft should be harvested at this point. The graft should be fashioned into a trapezoid with the largest portion placed superolaterally.
7. The osteotomy site can be fixed with a 2-hole semitubular plate.
8. After completion of osteotomy fixation, the foot should be assessed intraoperatively to judge whether additional procedures are needed.

Immediate postoperative care
A short-leg walking cast is applied with appropriate molding to hold correction. Patient may bear weight as tolerated.

Rehabilitation and recovery
The child should remain in a cast until the osteotomy is healed (usually 8–10 weeks). Patients may bear weight fully after the cast is removed. Arch supports or a supramalleolar orthosis may be needed in some children for additional comfort. No specific physical therapy protocol is needed after this operation.

Subtalar Fusion

Subtalar fusion should be considered in older children with severe planovalgus collapse. This procedure should not be undertaken on very young children, because it may decrease hindfoot growth.[9] Subtalar fusion can also be performed together with lateral column lengthening in children who are nonambulatory or with severe deformity.

Preoperative planning
Weight-bearing radiographs of the ankle and foot help to judge the severity of deformity and collapse. Subtalar fusion is indicated in children who are minimally ambulatory or nonambulatory with poor motor control and severe planovalgus deformity. Fusing the subtalar joint increases stress on adjacent joints and can lead to degeneration of function over time in high-functioning patients. Any additional areas of deformity noted on preoperative examination or radiographs must be addressed.

Patient positioning
The patient is positioned supine on a radiolucent table with proximal tourniquet applied.

Surgical approach and procedure
1. Skin incision is similar to that described for lateral calcaneal lengthening (curvilinear incision from anterior border of lateral malleolus to anterior aspect of peroneus brevis).
2. Dissection is carried out anterior to peroneus brevis, and subperiosteal dissection is used to identify the borders of the sinus tarsi. It is critical that all soft tissue in the sinus tarsi be removed to allow for appropriate visualization of the anterior, middle, and posterior facets. The capsule of the calcaneocuboid joint should be the distal extent of the dissection (see **Fig. 2**A).
3. Anterior and middle facet cartilage is denuded with a curette or osteotome, taking care not to remove any bone. No cartilage should be removed from the medial or lateral aspects of the posterior facet to avoid loss of height.[9]
4. A curvilinear medial incision is then made from the anterior tibialis insertion to the anteromedial aspect of the medial malleolus.
5. The talonavicular joint and the talar neck are exposed (**Fig. 3**A).
6. A guidewire in inserted through the anteromedial aspect of the talar neck so it will traverse the neck at a 45° angle (**Fig. 3**B). The starting point should be about 1 cm proximal to the cartilage on the talar head.
7. The subtalar joint should then be reduced, and the guidewire is advanced transversely so that it catches the anterior facet. The exit point of the pin in the inferior calcaneus should be 5 mm posterior to the calcaneocuboid joint.
8. Bone graft is placed into the sinus tarsi.
9. Before cannulated screw placement, the position of the hindfoot should be confirmed to ensure appropriate alignment. The talocalcaneal angle should be between 30° and 40°.
10. A cannulated screw can then be placed, fixing the hindfoot in position.
11. Sometimes a second screw in necessary in the older adolescent from the anterior aspect of the talus to the calcaneal tuberosity to provide extra stability.

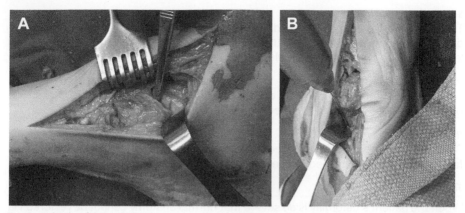

Fig. 3. Subtalar fusion. (*A*) Talonavicular joint. (*B*) Guidewire placed into talar neck for cannulated screw fixation.

12. The patient's forefoot should be reassessed to ensure that the first ray is not elevated.
13. If the navicular tuberosity is prominent, excision of the tuberosity should be considered. The tibialis posterior insertion can be sharply dissected, and the insertion is reattached with suture through the navicular once the prominence is removed.

Immediate postoperative care
A short leg cast is applied after wound closure and dressing. The patient is allowed to weight bear as tolerated in the cast. The cast is worn for 6 weeks.

Rehabilitation and recovery
No specific rehabilitation protocol is need after this procedure, and the child may resume their normal physical therapy routine. Orthotics are typically not needed postoperatively.

Equinovarus Foot Correction

Equinovarus deformity is significantly less common in children with cerebral palsy than planovalgus deformity. Hemiplegics with increasing deformity are candidates for operative intervention. As the deformity becomes more rigid, children can put more stress on the lateral aspect of the foot, causing callosities and pain. Surgical options for patients without fixed heel varus include surgery to tibialis anterior, surgery to tibialis posterior, or both.

Preoperative planning
Preoperative gait analysis is a helpful adjunct to thorough clinical examination to determine the most effective surgical management. EMG analysis of both the anterior tibialis and posterior tibialis should be obtained. In patients with swing phase or early stance phase varus, the tibialis anterior tendon can be overactive and firing throughout the gait cycle. These patients are good candidates for anterior tibialis transfer. Patients with increased varus throughout stance are better candidates for posterior tibialis transfer.

Patient positioning
The patient is placed supine with proximal tourniquet.

Surgical approach and technique

The technique for both anterior and posterior tibialis transfers are discussed in great detail in Tendon Transfers around the Foot: When and Where, by Kuo and colleagues.[10] Please refer to this article for technique pearls.

Immediate postoperative care

The patient is placed in a short leg cast in slight overcorrection for 4 to 6 weeks. The patient may bear weight as tolerated.

Rehabilitation and recovery

Some patients are placed in a hinged ankle–foot orthosis after cast removal. The need for an orthosis is determined by the position of the foot and any residual deformity.

Triple Arthrodesis

When the patient's deformity is so severe that normal anatomy cannot be restored via the soft tissue and boney procedures already mentioned, triple arthrodesis should be considered.[11,12] The triple arthrodesis combines subtalar fusion, calcaneocuboid lengthening fusion, and repair of the medial column. The arthrodesis is performed sequentially. Hindfoot malalignment must first be addressed with subtalar fusion. Midfoot alignment is restored with the calcaneocuboid fusion. Finally, the forefoot is treated with talonavicular arthrodesis.[13]

Preoperative planning

The severe nature of the patient's deformity can be assessed on clinical examination and by weight-bearing radiographs.

Patient positioning

The patient is placed supine on a radiolucent operating table. A tourniquet is placed on the upper thigh. A small bump can be placed under the ipsilateral buttocks to allow for better lateral visualization if needed.

Surgical approach and technique

1. The subtalar joint is exposed and fused as described in the subtalar arthrodesis section.
2. The calcaneocuboid joint is then exposed through the distal end of the incision made for the subtalar fusion.
3. The capsule of the calcaneocuboid joint is opened, and the cartilage on the cuboid is removed with a curette.
4. The cartilage on the calcaneal side of the joint can be removed in a direction perpendicular to the longitudinal axis of the forefoot with an oscillating saw or an osteotome.
5. A laminar spreader or Cobb elevators can now be used to open the calcaneocuboid joint (**Fig. 4**).
6. A bone graft (either autograft or allograft) should be made into a trapezoid and placed with its widest portion superiorly.
7. A semitubular plate is used to fix the bone graft in place.
8. Attention is then turned to the medial column. An incision is made along the anterior aspect of the talonavicular joint to the level of the first metatarsal.
9. Using sharp dissection, the talonavicular joint is opened.
10. If a large tuberosity is seen on the navicular, this can removed using the aforementioned technique.
11. The medial side should be carefully assessed for medial instability. The cartilage of the joints found to be unstable is then removed for planned fusion (most commonly the talonavicular joint and the navicular–medial cuneiform joint).

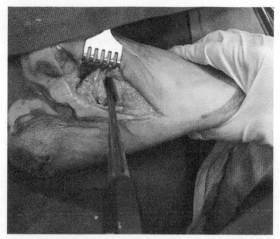

Fig. 4. Triple arthrodesis. Opening of calcaneocuboid joint for fusion.

12. Each planned fusion site (site of instability) should be opened sequentially to correct the deformity.
13. A bone graft is inserted to elevate the first ray and correct the deformity.
14. The fusion sites can be fixed with a plate and screw construct.

Immediate postoperative care
A short leg cast should be worn for 8 to 12 weeks depending on healing. The patient may bear weight as tolerated.

Rehabilitation and recovery
Full weight bearing can be continued once out of casts. The patient can return to their preexisting physical therapy regimen.

Clinical Results in the Literature

Equinus contracture
Equinus contracture is the most common foot and ankle deformity in children with cerebral palsy.[14] Many studies in the literature discuss both operative and nonoperative treatment, and various surgical techniques have been described. Many studies of equinus treatment caution against operative treatment in young children owing to fears regarding the high risk of recurrence and unpredictability of results.[15,16] Thus, the popularity of nonoperative measures such as orthotics and botulinum toxin injection have increased, leading to an increased age at index procedure. A recent systematic review by Shore and colleagues[17] looked at various patient and surgical factors in the literature that may affect outcomes. Because many studies on treatment of equinus are retrospective case series, it is difficult to make recommendations regarding the superiority of 1 technique or protocol over another. The authors concluded that randomized, controlled trials would be helpful to evaluate the effectiveness of different techniques. Regardless of the surgical technique used, most authors agree that overlengthening and occurrence of calcaneus deformity does have a negative effect on outcomes.

Ankle valgus
Ankle valgus has not been reported as an isolated lesion driving deformity, but is found in concert with other deformities such as the planovalgus foot. Thus, treatment of

ankle valgus should be included as only 1 tool in overall management of deformity. Medial epiphysiodesis screws have shown good results in a variety of pathologies,[18,19] but have not been studied extensively for patients with cerebral palsy. Much like ankle valgus from other etiologies, epiphysiodesis can be used in young children to guide their growth into a more neutral position.[9]

Lateral column lengthening and subtalar fusion

Planovalgus deformity is very common in children with cerebral palsy. Surgical treatment is undertaken if deformity progresses, gait is impacted, or the child has an increase in pain or shoe wear difficulty. Various techniques for reestablishing more normal anatomy have been described. Initially, isolated lateral column lengthening was described as ineffective for children with spastic deformity.[20] More recent studies have shown lateral column lengthening to be beneficial in higher functioning patients with less severe deformity.[21] A recent retrospective review of 78 patients who had undergone either lateral column lengthening or subtalar fusion showed that both procedures were effective, provided that the appropriate procedure was chosen based on the deformity.[5] This study is in keeping with others in the literature, who recommend subtalar fusion for more significant deformity in lower demand patients.[5,22]

Tendon transfers for equinovarus deformity

Spastic equinovarus deformity occurs more often in hemiplegics. As the drivers of the deformity can be complex, preoperative gait analysis with EMG,[23] kinematic analysis, and pedobarographs can assist in picking the correct procedure to ameliorate deformity. Posterior tibialis transfer for treatment of spastic varus deformity was described by Green and colleagues,[24] and the authors found good results in hemiplegics. Fractional lengthening of the posterior tibialis has been reported with good results and no patients with overcorrection.[25] Some authors prefer split transfers of the posterior tibialis in high-functioning hemiplegics and myofascial lengthening in diplegics.[9] However, there is not enough literature to draw conclusions regarding the most effective procedure. The consensus among authors on this topic is that overlengthening is to be avoided and can lead to planovalgus deformity. Split anterior tibialis transfers have yielded good results when performed on appropriate patients (those with EMG indicating anterior tibialis overactivity).[26] The most commonly described complication of split transfers has been deformity recurrence, which emphasizes the need to have a full understanding of the deformity before embarking on surgical treatment.

SUMMARY

Foot and ankle deformities in children with cerebral palsy can be effectively treated with surgery. Surgery should be considered in patients with significant deformity and those who have pain or difficulty with orthotic and shoe wear. Equinus contracture of both gastrocnemius and soleus can be treated with open tendoachilles lengthening. Ankle valgus of greater than $10°$ can be treated with medial epiphysiodesis. Pes planovalgus and equinus deformities are the most common deformity in children with cerebral palsy. In good ambulators with mild to moderate deformity, lateral column lengthening alone can be sufficient. Subtalar fusion is often combined with lateral column lengthening in patients with severe deformity and are nonambulatory. Equinovarus is more commonly seen in hemiplegic patients and this deformity can usually be treated with tendon transfers alone (anterior tibialis vs posterior tibialis) provided that heel varus is not fixed. Triple arthrodesis is an option in children with severe degenerative changes. It is important to address all aspects of the child's pathology at the time of surgical correction.

REFERENCES

1. Narayanan UG. Management of children with ambulatory cerebral palsy: an evidence-based review. J Pediatr Orthop 2012;32(Suppl 2):S172–81.
2. Bennet GC, Rang M, Jones D. Varus and valgus deformities of the foot in cerebral palsy. Dev Med Child Neurol 1982;24:499–503.
3. Perry J. Gait analysis: normal and pathologic function. Thorofare (NJ): Slack; 1992.
4. Rethlefsen SA, Kay RM. Transverse plane gait problems in children with cerebral palsy. J Pediatr Orthop 2013;33(4):422–30.
5. Kadhim M, Holmes L, Church C, et al. Pes planovalgus deformity surgical correction in ambulatory children with cerebral palsy. J Child Orthop 2012;6(3):217–27.
6. Miller F. Knee, leg, and foot. In: Miller F, editor. Cerebral palsy. New York: Springer; 2005. p. 667–802.
7. Driscoll MD, Linton J, Sullivan E, et al. Medial malleolar screw versus tension-band plate hemiepiphysiodesis for ankle valgus in the skeletally immature. J Pediatr Orthop 2014;34(4):441–6.
8. Bayhan IA, Yıldırım T, Beng K, et al. Medial malleolar screw hemiepiphysiodesis for ankle valgus in children with spina bifida. Acta Orthop Belg 2014;80(3):414–8.
9. Miller F. Surgical techniques. In: Miller F, editor. Cerebral palsy. New York: Springer; 2005. p. 865–1024.
10. Kuo KN, Wu K, Krzak JJ, et al. Tendon transfers around the foot: when and where. J Foot Ankle Surg 2015, in press.
11. Bishay SN. Single-event multilevel acute total correction of complex equinocavovarus deformity in skeletally mature patients with spastic cerebral palsy hemiparesis. J Foot Ankle Surg 2013;52(4):481–5.
12. Trehan SK, Ihekweazu UN, Root L. Long-term outcomes of triple arthrodesis in cerebral palsy patients. J Pediatr Orthop 2015;35(7):751–5.
13. Rathjen KE, Mubarak SJ. Calcaneal-cuboid-cuneiform osteotomy for the correction of valgus foot deformities in children. J Pediatr Orthop 1998;18(6):775–82.
14. Silver CM, Simon SD. Gastrocnemius-muscle recession (Silfverskiold operation) for spastic equinus deformity in cerebral palsy. J Bone Joint Surg Am 1959;41:1021–8.
15. Borton DC, Walker K, Pirpiris M, et al. Isolated calf lengthening in cerebral palsy. Outcome analysis of risk factors. J Bone Joint Surg Br 2001;83:364–70.
16. Banks HH. The management of spastic deformities of the foot and ankle. Clin Orthop Relat Res 1977;122:70–6.
17. Shore BJ, White N, Graham HK. Surgical correction of equinus deformity in children with cerebral palsy: a systemic review. J Child Orthop 2010;4(4):277–90.
18. Beals RK. The treatment of ankle valgus by surface epiphysiodesis. Clin Orthop 1991;(266):162–9.
19. Davids JR, Valadie AL, Ferguson RL, et al. Surgical management of ankle valgus in children: use of transphyseal medial malleolar screw. J Pediatr Orthop 1997;17:3–8.
20. Evans D. Calcaneo-valgus deformity. J Bone Joint Surg Br 1975;57:270–8.
21. Mosca VS. Calcaneal lengthening for valgus deformity of the hindfoot. Results in children who had severe, symptomatic flatfoot and skewfoot. J Bone Joint Surg Am 1995;77:500–12.
22. Dogan A, Zorer G, Mumcuoglu EI, et al. A comparison of two different techniques in the surgical treatment of flexible pes planovalgus: calcaneal lengthening and extra-articular subtalar arthrodesis. J Pediatr Orthop B 2009;18:167–75.

23. Renders A, Detrembleur C, Rossillon R. Contribution of electromyographic analysis of the walking habits of children with spastic foot in cerebral palsy: a preliminary study. Rev Chir Orthop Reparatrice Appar Mot 1997;83:259–64.

24. Green NE, Griffin PP, Shiavi R. Split posterior tibial tendon transfer in spastic cerebral palsy. J Bone Joint Surg Am 1983;65:748–54.

25. Ruda R, Frost H. Cerebral palsy. Spastic varus and forefoot adductus, treated by intramuscular posterior tibial tendon lengthening. Clin Orthop 1971;79:61–70.

26. Hoffer MM, Reisweig JA, Garrett MM, et al. The split anterior tibial transfer in cerebral palsied patients with spastic equinovarus deformity. J Pediatr Orthop 1985;5:432–4.

Tarsal Coalitions – Calcaneonavicular Coalitions

Stephanie J. Swensen, MD[a],*, Norman Y. Otsuka, MD[b,c]

KEYWORDS

- Tarsal coalition • Calcaneonavicular coalition • Pes planus • Resection

KEY POINTS

- Calcaneonavicular coalitions are aberrant osseous, cartilaginous, or fibrous unions between the calcaneal and navicular bones.
- Calcaneonavicular coalitions comprise the majority of tarsal coalitions and may be either congenital or acquired.
- Patients typically present between 8 and 12 years of age with complaints of vague foot pain and often a history of recurrent ankle sprains.
- Plain radiographs are the initial step in evaluation and advanced imaging modalities are useful for preoperative planning, identifying nonosseous calcaneonavicular coalitions, and degenerative changes within the foot.
- Treatment is indicated for painful coalitions and successful outcomes have been demonstrated with resection of calcaneonavicular coalitions.

INTRODUCTION

Calcaneonavicular coalitions are an important cause of adolescent foot pain and deformity. The congenital condition is characterized by an aberrant osseous, cartilaginous, or fibrinous union of the calcaneal and navicular bones. Calcaneonavicular coalitions are the most common form of tarsal coalitions identified within epidemiologic studies.[1] A thorough understanding of this clinically significant entity is important for restoring joint motion and preventing long-term disability.

HISTORY

Tarsal coalitions are an ancient concept and were first described formally by Buffon in 1796.[2] Cruveillhier is credited with providing the first anatomic description of

The authors have nothing to disclose.
[a] Department of Orthopaedic Surgery, New York University Hospital for Joint Diseases, 301 East 17th Street, New York, NY 10003, USA; [b] Pediatric Orthopaedics, The Children's Hospital at Montefiore, 3415 Brainbridge Ave., Bronx, NY 10457, USA; [c] Orthopaedic Surgery and Pediatrics, Albert Einstein College of Medicine, 1300 Morris Park Ave., Bronx, NY 10461, USA
* Corresponding author.
E-mail address: stephanie.swensen@nyumc.org

calcaneonavicular coalitions in 1829.[3] In a landmark study in 1948, Harris and Beath were the first to identify tarsal coalition as a cause of a painful, rigid flatfoot.[4]

EPIDEMIOLOGY

The overall incidence of calcaneonavicular coalitions is highly variable within the literature. The most commonly cited prevalence of tarsal coalitions is 1%.[1,5,6] However, this value is widely considered to be a gross underestimate of the true prevalence, given that many calcaneonavicular coalitions are asymptomatic. Additionally, the non-osseous subtypes of coalitions are not readily visible on plain radiographs and often remain undiagnosed.[5] Cadaveric and advanced imaging studies indicate the prevalence of tarsal coalitions to be as high as 13%.[1,5-7] Before the development of computed tomography (CT) and MRI, Pfitzner's cadaveric study of 520 subjects in 1896 was considered to be the most accurate representation of the true incidence of tarsal coalitions in the general population, with a reported incidence of 6%.[6,8] A more recent radiologic study by Lysack and Fenton[7] found a 5.6% incidence of calcaneonavicular coalitions in particular. These studies also demonstrated that tarsal coalitions are bilateral in 50% to 68% of cases.[1,9]

An equal sex distribution is generally accepted; however, a number of studies indicate a slight male predominance. Conway and Cowell[10] identified tarsal coalitions in 4 times as many men than women and Menz and colleagues[11] noted that operations are performed for tarsal coalitions in men at a rate 1.5 times that of women.

ETIOLOGY

Calcaneonavicular coalitions may be either congenital or acquired. Tarsal coalitions can develop as a result of trauma, surgery, arthritis, infection, and neoplasia.[5,9] The majority of calcaneonavicular coalitions are congenital, as proposed by Leboucq in 1890. The coalitions are believed to develop owing to failure of embryonic mesenchymal differentiation and segmentation.[12] Calcaneonavicular coalitions are inherited via an autosomal-dominant mode of inheritance with variable penetrance.[13,14] In a study of first-degree relatives of individuals with confirmed tarsal coalitions, Leonard found that the inheritance pattern is more complicated than simple Mendelian genetics because the location of the coalition (talocalcaneal or calcaneonavicular) was not consistent among generations.[5,13] Calcaneonavicular coalitions are also known to be associated with other congenital disorders, including fibular hemimelia, symphalagism, arthrogryposis, Apert syndrome, and Nievergelt–Pearlman syndrome.[14,15]

CLASSIFICATION

Calcaneonavicular coalitions are typically classified morphologically as osseous, cartilaginous, or fibrinous. Upasani and colleagues[16] recently proposed a classification scheme based on the appearance of the coalition and the relationship to adjacent tarsal bones on the plantar view. The authors analyzed calcaneonavicular coalitions using multiplanar 3-dimensional CT and categorized the coalitions into 4 major types: type I (form fruste), type II (fibrous), type III (cartilaginous), and type IV (osseous). Forme fruste variants were noted to have cortical irregularities at the tip of the calcaneus or an ossicle present between the calcaneus and navicular bones in addition to slight blunting of the cuboid. Fibrous coalitions included further blunting of the cuboid extension and narrowing of the nonossified gap between the calcaneus and navicular bones. Type III coalitions had near-complete or cartilaginous fusion between the bones and a distinct "squaring-off" of the cuboid bone. Type IV coalitions have complete osseous fusion between the calcaneal and navicular bones and are characterized by a dramatic change in the shape of the cuboid bone.

CLINICAL PRESENTATION

Calcaneonavicular coalitions most commonly present between 8 and 12 years of age. The onset of symptoms is typically associated with the time of ossification of the coalition. During this period, the foot stiffens and the coalition alters the kinematics of the involved joint.[17] In their prospective study, Katayama and colleagues[18] directly correlated the onset of symptoms with progressive evidence of ossification on imaging. A histopathologic analysis of tarsal coalitions by Kumai and colleagues[19] found an absence of nerve fibers within coalition and hypothesized that the pain develops as a result of microfracturing at the coalition–bone interface, generating pain through the periosteal nerve fibers.[17]

Patients with calcaneonavicular coalitions classically present with vague foot pain that is worse with activity and improves with rest. The child may be reluctant to participate in physical activities and often becomes more sedentary. Patients report difficult walking on uneven surfaces and uncomfortable tightness of the calf. Calcaneonavicular coalitions are also frequently unmasked in the setting of minor trauma. Patients present with a history of an ankle or foot injury that fails to resolve. A history of recurrent ankle sprains should raise suspicion for the presence of a coalition.[20] The pain is typically diffuse, but can be localized frequently to the sinus tarsi with calcaneonavicular coaltions.[17]

Observation of the patient reveals an antalgic galt with decreased stance phase of the affected extremity and patient often have an out-toeing gait.[21] There is valgus alignment of the hindfoot in the standing position. Flattening of the medial longitudinal arch commonly develops as the distal joints overcompensate for the stiffness resulting from the coalition.[13] Although a flatfoot deformity is associated most commonly with calcaneonavicular coalitions, cavovarus deformities may also occur infrequently.[17,22] A single-leg heel raise test is used to assess the flexibility of the flat foot deformity. Patients with calcaneonavicular coalitions typically fail to reconstitute the arch of the foot, indicating a rigid hindfoot.

The finding of "peroneal spastic flat foot" was initially thought to be pathognomonic for tarsal coalition.[4] Peroneal spastic flat foot is characterized by hindfoot rigid valgus and forefoot abduction caused by spasms of the peroneal muscles. The peroneal tendons attempt to overcome the limited subtalar motion and the peroneal muscles reflexively contract with inversion of the hindfoot.[23] However, peroneal spastic flat foot may be caused by a number of other pathologies, including rheumatoid arthritis, osteoid osteoma, and hindfoot injury, and is therefore not definitively indicative of tarsal coalition.[24]

Tenderness to palpation may be elicited directly over and distal to the anterior process of the calcaneus in calcaneonavicular coalitions.[22] Range of motion testing reveals diminished motion of the subtalar joint with a decrease in inversion and eversion. Comparison should be made with the contralateral foot, but frequently the findings are present on both sides.

IMAGING

The initial diagnostic evaluation of all patients with a suspected calcaneonavicular coalition begins with plain radiographs. Three views of the feet are obtained: anteroposterior, lateral, and 45° oblique weight-bearing views. The 45° oblique view, as described by Slomann in 1921,[25] is the best view for imaging calcaneonavicular coalitions on radiographs. This view has been found to demonstrate the presence of a calcaneonavicular coalition in 90% to 100% of cases.[26,27] Careful evaluation for the presence of a coalition is often difficult on plain radiographs owing to significant overlap of the tarsal bones, but a few distinct signs have been described to aid in diagnosis. The "anteater sign" is diagnostic for calcaneonavicular coalitions. The sign was described initially on oblique radiographs, but is also easily visible on lateral views.[10,28,29] The anterior process of the calcaneus is normally triangular, but becomes elongated with coalitions and the tip is squared like the snout of an anteater. One study by Crim and Kjeldsberg[29] demonstrated a sensitivity of 72% and 90% specificity of the "anteater sign" on lateral radiographs. Talar beaking may also be identified on lateral radiographs.[26] The elongated navicular sign or "reverse anteater sign" is another radiographic sign described for calcaneonavicular coalitions and is visible on anteroposterior radiographs of the foot.[28] The lateral margin of the navicular bone normally aligns with the head of the talus. The morphology of the navicular bone is altered in calcaneonavicular coalitions and the navicular extends laterally. This sign was originally reported to have a sensitivity of 50% and a specificity of 100%[29]; however, subsequent studies reported a very low sensitivity of 18%.[30] Additionally, the plain radiographs should be analyzed for evidence of adjacent joint arthrosis, which changes the options for surgical management.

CT is the gold standard imaging technique to evaluate calcaneonavicular coalitions. This imaging modality offers a more precise depiction of the location and size of the calcaneonavicular coalition and is also effective for identifying concomitant coalitions. CT is also useful for confirming degenerative changes at other joints for preoperative planning. Herzenberg and colleagues[31] demonstrated the ability of CT to identify both osseous and nonosseous talocalcaneal coalitions[27] and Upasani and colleagues[16] similarly showed the superiority of CT for visualizing calcaneonavicular coalitions. Cross-sections of 3 mm or less are optimal for identifying calcaneonavicular bars because the bars are often obliquely oriented and can be mistaken for normal bone on some cross sectional views. Disadvantages of CT include increased radiation exposure and lower sensitivity for detecting nonosseous coalitions.[32]

MRI is a particularly useful modality for evaluating nonosseous calcaneonavicular coalitions. The sagittal and axial views are best for visualizing these coalitions. Nalaboff and colleagues[30] suggest that the subtle signs of calcaneonavicular coalitions, such as the reverse anteater, are better seen on MRI than plain film. MRI has the ability to show the density and characteristic of the bridging material in detail. Additionally, MRI has the benefit of evaluating concomitant soft tissue pathology and bone marrow edema.[8] Similar to CT, the modality can confirm the presence of early joint degeneration. In a blinded comparison of MRI and CT of 15 identified coalitions, Emery and colleagues[33] demonstrated a high rate of agreement among MRI and CT for detecting tarsal coalition. Another recent study by Guignand and colleagues[34] evaluated 19 patients who underwent surgical treatment for calcaneonavicular tarsal coalitions and had both CT and MRI. In the study, CT missed 4 cases (2 cartilaginous and 2 fibrous), which were both identified on MRI, therefore leading the authors to conclude that MRI is the most effective means of precise diagnosis. Furthermore, although MRI has the disadvantage of high cost, MRI does not expose the growing patient to radiation.

TREATMENT

Treatment is only indicated for painful coalitions because there has yet to be evidence to demonstrate that asymptomatic calcaneonavicular coalitions cause significant disability.[35] The type of treatment indicated for symptomatic calcaneonavicular coalitions depends on a number of factors, including the severity of symptoms and the presence of degenerative changes within the foot.

Nonoperative treatment is indicated as the first line of treatment for all coalitions. Initial treatments include activity modification, nonsteroidal antiinflammatory drugs, flat bottom orthoses, and cast immobilization. A trial of a short leg walking cast with the hindfoot in neutral for 4 to 6 weeks should be attempted in all cases. An estimated 30% of patients remain pain free after removal of the cast.[27,35] However, calcaneonavicular coalitions are less likely to respond to nonoperative treatment than talonavicular coalitions.

Operative management is considered for all patients with recurrent or persistent pain after conservative treatment. Surgical options include resection of the coalition or arthrodesis. Additionally, if a pes planovalgus deformity is seen in association with a calcaneonavicular coalition, then an Evans or medializing calcaneal osteotomy may be considered at the same time as the resection.[36] Badgley was the first to describe surgical resection of calcaneonavicular coalition in 1927.[37] Cowell[38] later modified the original technique by adding interposition of the extensor digitorum brevis (EDB) to the resection. Current options for interposition after coalition resection include EDB muscle, bone wax applied to cancellous surfaces, fat, and no material. A major contraindication to calcaneonavicular coalition resection is degenerative arthritis. Patients with evidence of arthritis on preoperative imaging are indicated for triple arthrodesis.

OPERATIVE TECHNIQUE
Preoperative Planning

Before surgery, it is imperative to determine if there are any additional coalitions or evidence of degenerative changes on imaging. Adequate characterization of the coalition must be performed, with determination of the size, depth, and nature of the coalition. Upasani and colleagues[16] emphasized the importance of preoperative imaging with 3-dimensional CT to avoid iatrogenic injury and to ensure complete excision of the coalition. Espinosa and colleagues[39] similarly proposed computer-aided CT analysis and reconstructions to help determine the spatial orientation of calcaneonavicular coalitions before surgery, given the high percentage of morphologic abnormalities of the anterior calcaneal facets. Thus, thorough evaluation of preoperative imaging is required before resection of the calcaneonavicular coalitions.

Positioning

- The patient is placed supine on a radiolucent table with a bump under the hip of the operative leg to provide slight internal rotation of the extremity.
- A sterile tourniquet is placed on the ipsilateral thigh.
- If fat autograft is to be obtained from the buttock, then the extremity is prepped to just above the gluteal crease. Alternatively, an additional abdominal site is prepped for harvesting of the fat autograft.

Operative Approach

- Key landmarks, including the anterior process of the calcaneus, the cuboid, the fifth metatarsal, and the peroneal tendons, are marked on the skin.[13,21,40]
- An oblique incision is made along the dorsolateral aspect of the foot extending from the anterior process of the calcaneus to the navicular (Ollier approach; **Fig. 1**). Care must be taken not to undermine the fragile tissue during this approach.
- Superiorly, expose the long extensor tendons and retract them medially without opening the sheaths.
- Expose and retract the peroneal tendons inferiorly.
- Identify and incise the inferior extensor retinaculum to expose the origin of the EDB.

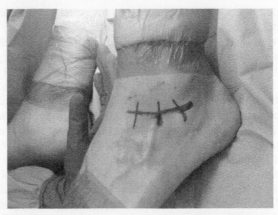

Fig. 1. An oblique incision is marked along the dorsolateral aspect of the foot, extending from the anterior process of the calcaneus to the navicular. (*Courtesy of* Dr Andrew Price, New York, NY.)

- Follow the EDB proximally to the sinus tarsi. Incise the fibrofatty tissue within the sinus tarsi to expose the origin of the EDB.
- Incise and reflect the origin of the EDB distally to expose the anterior process of the calcaneus and the calcaneonavicular coalition. Avoid extending the dissection into the calcaneocuboid joint.

Operative Procedure

- Remove a trapezoidal piece of bone under direct fluoroscopic assistance with a 0.25- or 0.5-inch osteotome (**Fig. 2**).[13,21,40]
  - The first cut is made at the medial aspect of the anterior process of the calcaneus, angled 40° to 60° from the vertical and directed medially toward the lateral aspect of the navicular. Take caution to avoid damaging the talar head with the osteotome.
  - The second cut is made at the lateral aspect of the navicular and directed toward the same point as the first cut.
- Remove the excised piece of bone and use a pituitary or Kerrison rongeur to resect the remaining portions of the coalition (**Fig. 3**).

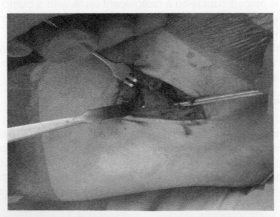

Fig. 2. The long extensor tendons are retracted medially and the peroneal tendons are retracted inferiorly to expose the calcaneonavicular coalition. (*Courtesy of* Dr Andrew Price, New York, NY.)

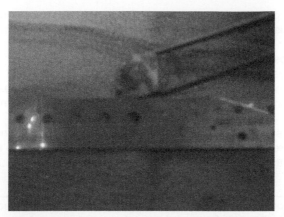

Fig. 3. The trapezoidal piece of bone is excised with a 0.25- or 0.5-inch osteotome. (*Courtesy of* Dr Andrew Price, New York, NY.)

- Ensure that enough bone is removed to create a visible space (1 × 1 cm) between the calcaneus and the navicular. The most common error is to excise too little bone from the plantar–medial corner of the bar.
- Confirm complete resection on fluoroscopy. On the oblique view, adequate resection has been performed when a line drawn along the lateral border of the talar neck falls adjacent to the lateral-most aspect of the navicular and another line drawn along the medial aspect of the calcaneus lies adjacent to the medial border of the cuboid.
- Check hindfoot motion.
- A thin layer of a hemostatic agent, such as FloSeal, bone wax, or fibrin glue, is applied to the area of resection[41] (**Fig. 4**).
- Fat autograft interposition:
  - Harvesting of the fat autograft may be performed before or after resection of the calcaneonavicular coalition. A transverse incision is made in the gluteal crease of the operative leg and a piece of subcutaneous fat (approximately 2 cm) is removed.

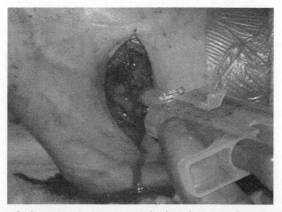

Fig. 4. A thin layer of a hemostatic agent is applied to the area of resection. (*Courtesy of* Dr Andrew Price, New York, NY.)

- ○ The fat is placed directly into the excised calcaneonavicular coalition.
- ○ The EDB is then sutured back to its origin to restore the normal contour of the foot.
- EDB interposition:
  - ○ Heavy, absorbable sutures are placed through the proximal end of the EDB and the ends of the sutures are passed through Keith needles.
  - ○ The Keith needles are passed through the space and exit the medial side of the foot.
  - ○ The sutures are then passed through a piece of sterile felt and a button. The sutures are then tied over the button to draw the muscle into the gap created between the anterior process of the calcaneus and the navicular.

Closure

- The tourniquet is released and adequate hemostasis is achieved.
- The wound is closed in layers with absorbable sutures and either an absorbable subcuticular suture or nonabsorbable nylon sutures for skin.
- A short leg splint is applied.

REHABILITATION AND RECOVERY

Postoperatively, patients remain non–weight-bearing in a short leg cast or splint for 3 weeks. Patients are then transitioned to weight-bearing as tolerated in a walking boot. Subtalar range of motion exercises are begun with the removal of the short leg cast. Physical therapy may be provided if there is significant stiffness to assist with range of motion, strengthening, and proprioception training.[40] Patients are typically allowed to return to full activities if comfortable at 6-week postoperative visit. Radiographs are then obtained at the 3-month, 6-month, and 1-year postoperative visits to assess resection gap.

COMPLICATIONS

Superficial infections and wound breakdown are the most common complications associated with operative resection for calcaneonavicular coalitions[5]. Injury of the adjacent cartilage during resection may also result in persistent pain and early degenerative changes after surgery. The talonavicular capsule may also be violated during the surgery, which can result in subluxation of the navicular on the talus, thereby further altering foot and ankle biomechanics. Failure of complete resection would be characterized by continued pain and loss of motion. Triple arthrodesis can be performed as a salvage procedure for failed operative resection.

CLINICAL RESULTS IN THE LITERATURE

The overall results of calcaneonavicular coalition resection procedures are very good, with approximately 80% to 90% acceptable results.[13] Cowell[24] suggested that the best long-term results after excision are to be expected in patients younger than 14 years of age. Early studies of resection procedures by Mitchell and Gibson[42] reported that excision without interposition material is an acceptable alternative to arthrodesis in patients with symptomatic calcaneonavicular coalitions. However, bone recurrence was documented in 67% of patients in this study, thus raising the questions as to the need for interposition material.

The evidence for the ideal interpositional material remains controversial within the literature. Moyes and colleagues[43] performed a retrospective review of 17 resected calcaneonavicular coalitions comparing EDB transposition with no soft tissue interposition. The authors found recurrence of the coalition only within the cohort with no soft tissue interposition. Cohen and colleagues[44] observed wound dehiscence in 3 out of 6 adult patients who underwent EDB interposition. Other adverse outcomes associated with EDB interposition include prominence of the calcaneocuboid joint owing to repositioning of EDB origin, which results in friction with shoe wear and poor cosmesis.[40] Mubarak and colleagues[40] recently reported the significant advantages of using fat as the interposition material. The study demonstrated lower reossification and reoperation rates with fat graft interposition compared with prior reports of EDB interposition. The cadaveric component of Mubarak's study also demonstrated that the EDB is only able to fill 64% of the resected gap, leaving approximately 10 mm of the plantar gap unfilled. Therefore, resection of calcaneonavicular coalitions with fat interposition is an effective method of surgical treatment for this condition.

REFERENCES

1. Stormont DM, Peterson HA. The relative incidence of tarsal coalition. Clin Orthop Relat Res 1983;(181):28–36.
2. Buffon GLL, Comte de. Histoire naturelle, generale et particuliere, Tome 3. Paris (France): Imprimieri Royale; 1769. p. 47.
3. Cruveilhier J. Anatomie pathologieque du corps humain. [Pathologic anatomy of the human corps] [in French]. Paris (France): Tome I. J. B. Bailliere; 1820.
4. Harris RI, Beath T. Etiology of peroneal spastic flat foot. J Bone Joint Surg 1948; 30:624–34.
5. Zaw H, Calder JDF. Tarsal coalitions. Foot Ankle Clin N Am 2010;15:349–64.
6. Pfitzner W. Die Variationem im Aufbau des Fusskelets. Morphologisches Arbeiten 1896;6:245–527.
7. Lysack JT, Fenton PV. Variations in calcaneonavicular morphology demonstrated with radiography. Radiology 2004;230:493–7.
8. Kernbach KJ. Tarsal coalitions: etiology, diagnosis, imaging, and stigmata. Clin Podiatr Med Surg 2010;27:105–17.
9. Mosier KM, Asher M. Tarsal coalitions and peroneal spastic flatfoot. A review. J Bone Joint Surg Am 1984;66:976–84.
10. Conway JJ, Cowell HR. Tarsal coalition: clinical significance and roentgenographic demonstration. Radiology 1969;92(4):799–811.
11. Menz HB, Gilheany MF, Landorf KB. Foot and ankle surgery in Australia: a descriptive analysis of the Medicare Benefits Schedule database, 1997-2006. J Foot Ankle Res 2008;15(1):1–10.
12. Leboucq H. De la Soudure Congenitale de Certains Os du Tarse. Bull Acad R Med Belg 1890;4:103–12.
13. Mosca VS. Tarsal coalitions. In: Weinstein SL, Flynn JM, editors. Lovell and Winter's pediatric orthopaedics. 7th edition. Philadelphia: Lippincott Williams & Wilkins; 2014. p. 1504–15.
14. Leonard MA. The inheritance of tarsal coalition and its relationship to spastic flat foot. J Bone Joint Surg 1974;56-B:520–6.
15. Grogan DP, Holt GR, Ogden JA. Talocalcaneal coalition patients who have fibular hemimelia or proximal femoral focal deficiency. A comparison of the radiographic and pathological findings. J Bone Joint Surg Am 1994;76: 1363–70.

16. Upasani VV, Chambers RC, Mubarak SJ. Analysis of calcaneonavicular coalition using multi-planar three-dimensional computed tomography. J Child Orthop 2008;2:301–7.

17. Lemley F, Berlet G, Hill K, et al. Current concepts review: tarsal coalitions. Foot Ankle Int 2006;27(12):1163–9.

18. Katayama T, Tanaka Y, Kadono K, et al. Talocalcaneal coalition: a case showing the ossification process. Foot Ankle Int 2005;26:490–3.

19. Kumai T, Takakura Y, Akiyama K, et al. Histopathological study of nonosseous tarsal coalitions. Foot Ankle Int 1998;19:525–31.

20. Snyder RB, Lipscomb AB, Johnston RK. The relationship of tarsal coalition to ankle sprains in athletes. Am J Sports Med 1981;9:313–7.

21. Demetracopoulos CA, Scher DM. Resection of calcaneonavicular coalition and fat autograft interposition. In: Kocher, Mininder S, Millis, et al, editors. Operative techniques: pediatric orthopaedic surgery. Philadelphia: Elsevier/Saunders; 2011. p. 604–14.

22. Stuecker RD, Bennet JT. Tarsal coalition presenting as a pes cavovarus deformity: report of three cases and review of the literature. Foot Ankle 1993;14:540–4.

23. Bohn WHO. Tarsal coalition. Curr Opin Pediatr 2001;13:29–35.

24. Cowell HR. Talocalcaneal coalition and new causes of peroneal spastic flatfoot. Clin Orthop 1972;85:16–22.

25. Slomann HC. On coalition calcaneo-navicularis. J Orthop Surg 1921;3:586–602.

26. Newman JS, Newberg AH. Congenital tarsal coalition: multimodality evaluation with emphasis on CT and MR imaging. Radiographics 2000;20(2):321–2.

27. Jayakumar S, Cowell HR. Rigid flatfoot. Clin Orthop 1977;122:77–84.

28. Crim J. Imaging of tarsal coalition. Radiol Clin N Am 2008;46:1017–26.

29. Crim JR, Kjeldsberg KM. Radiographic diagnosis of tarsal coalition. AJR Am J Roentgenol 2004;182(2):323–8.

30. Nalaboff KM, Schweitzer ME. MRI of tarsal coalition: frequency, distribution, and innovative signs. Bull NYU Hosp Jt Dis 2008;66(1):14–21.

31. Herzenberg JE, Goldner JL, Martinez S, et al. Computerized tomography of talocalcaneal tarsal coalition: a clinical and anatomic study. Foot Ankle 1986;6: 273–88.

32. Solomon LB, Ruhli FJ, Taylor J, et al. A dissection and computer tomograph study of tarsal coalitions in 100 cadaver feet. J Orthop Res 2003;21(2):352–8.

33. Emery KH, Bisset GS III, Johnson ND, et al. Tarsal coalition: a blinded comparison of MRI and CT. Pediatr Radiol 1998;28:612–6.

34. Guignand D, Journeau P, Mainard-Simard L, et al. Child calcaneonavicular coalitions: MRI diagnostic value in a 19-case series. Orthop Traumatol Surg Res 2011;97(1):67–72.

35. Mosca VS. Flexible flatfoot and tarsal coalition. In: Richards B, editor. Orthopaedic knowledge update: pediatrics. Rosemont (IL): American Academy of Orthopaedic Surgeons; 1996. p. 211.

36. Cass AD, Camasta CA. A review of tarsal coalition and pes planovalgus: clinical exam, imaging, and surgical planning. J Foot Ankle Surg 2010;49:274–93.

37. Badgley C. Coalitions of the calcaneus and the navicular. Arch Surg 1927;15: 75–88.

38. Cowell H. Extensor brevis arthroplasty. J Bone Joint Surg Am 1970;82:820.

39. Espinosa N, Dudda M, Andersen J, et al. Prediction of spatial orientation and morphology of calcaneonavicular coalitions. Foot Ankle Int 2008;29:205–12.

40. Mubarak SJ, Patel PN, Upasani VV, et al. Calcaneonavicular coalition: treatment by excision and fat graft. J Pediatr Orthop 2009;29:418–26.

41. Weatherall JM, Price AE. Fibrin glue as interposition graft for tarsal coalition. Am J Orthop (Belle Mead NJ) 2013;42(1):26–9.
42. Mitchell GP, Gibson JMC. Exclusion of calcaneonavicular bar for painful syasmotic flatfoot. J Bone Joint Surg Br 1967;49:281–7.
43. Moyes ST, Crawfurd EJP, Aichroth PM. The interposition of extensor digitorum brevis in the resection of calcaneonavicular bars. J Pediatr Orthop 1994;14: 387–8.
44. Cohen BE, Davis WH, Anderson RB. Success of calcaneonavicular coalition resection in the adult population. Foot Ankle Int 1996;17:569–72.

Talocalcaneal Coalitions

Joshua S. Murphy, MD[a], Scott J. Mubarak, MD[a,b],*

KEYWORDS

- Tarsal • Talocalcaneal • Coalition • Treatment • Pediatric

KEY POINTS

- Talocalcaneal coalitions present with complaints of flatfeet, foot or ankle pain after minor injury, or persistent ankle sprains.
- Physical examination findings: limited subtalar motion and prominence inferior to the medial malleolus.
- Use of computed topography (CT) scan is recommended for preoperative planning and confirmation of resection with intraoperative CT.
- Resection of talocalcaneal coalitions with fat-graft interposition has superior results to primary arthrodesis.
- Improved outcomes have been reported after resection with foot scores averaging 90/100 (AOFAS).

INTRODUCTION

Tarsal coalition was thought to be first described by Zuckerland in 1877.[1] In 1921, Sloman linked tarsal coalitions to rigid flatfeet.[1,2] Then, in 1994, Lateur and colleagues[3] described the "C" sign on a lateral foot radiograph, which they believed was indicative for a talocalcaneal coalition.

Tarsal coalitions are a result of failure of segmentation of the primitive mesenchyme during development, with further failure of formation of a normal joint.[4] The underlying inheritance pattern has been suggested to be autosomal dominant. Tarsal coalitions have a reported prevalence of 1% to 2%, with middle facet talocalcaneal coalitions (TCCs) making up 25% to 40% of tarsal coalitions, second only to calcaneonavicular coalitions.[5–8] Bilaterality has been reported in 50% of patients with TCCs.[4,9]

SIGNS AND SYMPTOMS

Tarsal coalitions typically cause stiffness of the subtalar joint and present between the ages of 8 and 16 years.[10] Patients with TCC tend to present slightly later than those

The authors have nothing to disclose.
[a] Department of Orthopedics, Rady Children's Hospital, 3030 Children's Way, Suite 410, San Diego, CA 92123, USA; [b] University of California San Diego, San Diego, CA 92093, USA
* Corresponding author.
E-mail address: smubarak@rchsd.org

with a calcaneonavicular coalition with activity-related hindfoot and/or midfoot pain. The timing tends to correspond with ossification of the tarsal bones.[11] Patients will often present with foot and/or ankle injuries, pain, or flatfeet. Gantsoudes and colleagues[12] reported their results on treatment of TCC and found that although pain was the most common presenting symptom, a significant number of patients presented after an injury, including ankle sprains and fracture.

PHYSICAL EXAMINATION

1. Limited subtalar motion if performed with the ankle in near neutral position.
2. Double medial malleolus sign: prominence palpated inferior to the medial malleolus, which represents the enlarged medial facet.

RADIOGRAPHIC EVALUATION

At our institution, we use the following 4 views on patients with stiffness and/or pain:

1. Standing anteroposterior bilateral feet
2. Standing lateral bilateral feet
3. 45° internal oblique X-ray to detect calcaneonavicular coalitions
4. Harris heel view to detect TCCs

Recently, Moraleda and Mubarak reported on the prevalence of the C sign on standing lateral foot films and its relationship to TCC. They concluded that a complete C sign is present in 15% of cases and likely indicates the presence of a TCC. The same study identified that an interrupted C sign is present in 77% of TCC cases. However, an interrupted C sign is also prevalent in 45% of flexible flat feet without a TCC.

Although these findings should heighten suspicion for pathology, treatment should be based on symptoms and physical examination, with diagnosis confirmed by computed tomography (CT) scan.

A CT scan can provide valuable data into the shape and size of the coalition for preoperative planning.[13,14]

PREOPERATIVE PLANNING

All patients receive a CT scan with 3-dimensional (3D) reconstruction for preoperative planning. As defined by the Tarsal Coalition Protocol in the radiology department at our institution, all patients are positioned supine on the examination table with both feet flat against a positioning box. The patients are scanned feet first, from the bottom of the feet proximally through the ankle joint.

Rozansky and colleagues[14] described a radiologic classification of 5 types of TCC based on CT 3D reconstruction: type I, linear coalitions (41%); type II, linear coalitions with a posterior hook (17%); type III, shingled coalitions (15%); type IV, complete osseous coalitions (11%); and type V, posterior coalitions (17%) (**Fig. 1**).

SURGICAL INDICATIONS

In the opinion of the Moraleda and colleagues[1], all symptomatic TCCs should undergo resection unless there are 2 coalitions or the TCCs are solid and very large. It is thought the underlying pathology will eventually lead to painful degenerative changes throughout the course of the patient's life. Casting for symptomatic relief has not routinely been used in our institution. However, it is the practice of some to incorporate a trial of nonoperative treatment before considering surgery. This includes a trial of immobilization in a short-leg walking cast for 2 to 4 weeks, followed by fitting for an orthosis. If the patient has pain

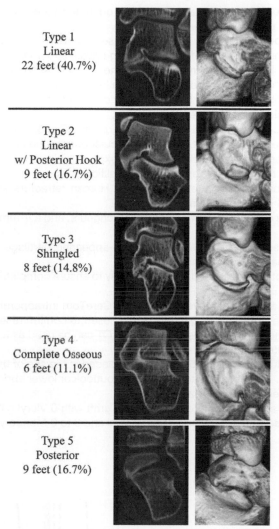

Type 1
Linear
22 feet (40.7%)

Type 2
Linear
w/ Posterior Hook
9 feet (16.7%)

Type 3
Shingled
8 feet (14.8%)

Type 4
Complete Osseous
6 feet (11.1%)

Type 5
Posterior
9 feet (16.7%)

Fig. 1. Talocalcaneal classification scheme. (*From* Rozansky A, Varley E, Mubarak SJ, et al. A radiologic classification of talocalcaneal coalitions based on 3D reconstruction. J Child Orthop 2010;4:130; with permission.)

relief with the cast, but recurs with the orthosis, the patient may be placed into a second cast. However, if this is not effective, surgery should be considered.[4]

PROCEDURE

Several techniques for operative management have been described for the treatment of TCCs. Earlier studies show successful treatment with arthrodesis, whereas more recently favorable outcomes have been reported with excision of the coalition.[12,15–17] Currently, symptomatic TCCs are treated with coalition resection and fat-graft interposition in our institution.[12] In this article, we discuss the senior author's preferred technique for resection of a TCC. The technique used is similar to that originally described by Olney and Asher.[18]

- Patient is positioned supine on a regular operating table with all bony prominences well padded.
- Leg is prepped and draped free with the use of a sterile tourniquet.
- Loupe magnification is helpful in identifying critical structures.
- A medial incision is made inferior to the medial malleolus over the bony bump caused by the coalition, and extending the length of the subtalar joint (**Fig. 2**).
- Sheaths of tibialis posterior (TP) and flexor digitorum longus (FDL) are identified and an incision made to open the sheaths.
- FDL is retracted inferior and TP retracted superior (**Fig. 3**). If a posterior hook or posterior coalition is present, the neurovascular bundle and flexor hallucis longus are also identified and protected. The flexor hallucis longus (FHL) is closely adherent to the posterior aspect of the coalition.
- Once the coalition is fully exposed, small Homan retractors are placed in the anterior and posterior facets (**Fig. 4**).
- Resection is completed with osteotomes, rongeurs, and a 4-mm high-speed bur (**Fig. 5**).
- Coalition resection continues until normal-appearing cartilage of the posterior facet is visualized (**Figs. 6** and **7**).
- Hindfoot motion is assessed intraoperatively to ensure complete resection of the coalition.
- In addition, an intraoperative CT scanner (CereTom intraoperative CT scanner; NeuroLogica Corporation, Danvers, MA) is used to confirm resection. If residual coalition is noted on intraoperative CT, the CT can be used as a guide to identify and complete the resection (**Fig. 8**).[19]
- At the conclusion of resection, fat graft is placed in the site of the previous excision (**Fig. 9**). The fat can be taken from the buttock or lower abdomen. Bone wax is then placed on bony surfaces.
- The tendon sheath is repaired over the fat graft with 0 Vicryl suture.
- Skin is closed with a 3-0 Vicryl deep dermal and 3 to 0 Monocryl superficial skin suture.

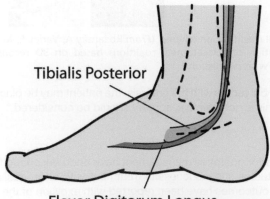

Tibialis Posterior

Flexor Digitorum Longus

Fig. 2. Incision is made just inferior to the medial malleolus, overlying the TP and FDL tendons. (*From* Gantsoudes GD, Roocroft JH, Mubarak SJ. Treatment of talocalcaneal coalitions. J Pediatr Orthop 2012;32:302; with permission.)

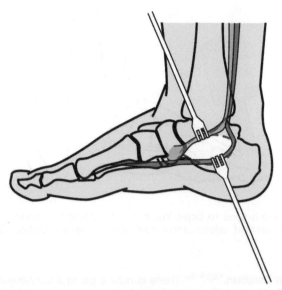

Fig. 3. TP is retracted anterior and FDL is retracted inferior. (*From* Gantsoudes GD, Roocroft JH, Mubarak SJ. Treatment of talocalcaneal coalitions. J Pediatr Orthop 2012;32:302; with permission.)

POSTOPERATIVE TREATMENT

All patients are placed in a short-leg cast and encouraged to begin weight bearing as tolerated immediately after surgery. The casts are removed at 3 weeks, and patients transition to a sturdy athletic shoe. They begin exercising and physical therapy to improve strength and range of motion on removal of the cast.[12]

CLINICAL RESULTS

The treatment for symptomatic TCCs has been widely reported in the literature, and has evolved from earlier recommendations of subtalar or triple arthrodeses[10,20–23]

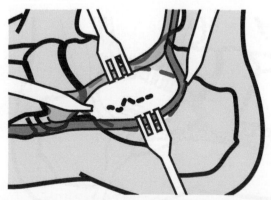

Fig. 4. Small Hohmann retractors are placed in the anterior and posterior facets to delineate the coalition and to mark the ends of the resection. (*From* Gantsoudes GD, Roocroft JH, Mubarak SJ. Treatment of talocalcaneal coalitions. J Pediatr Orthop 2012;32:302; with permission.)

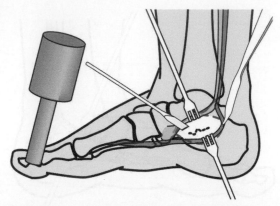

Fig. 5. An osteotome is used to begin the resection. (*From* Gantsoudes GD, Roocroft JH, Mubarak SJ. Treatment of talocalcaneal coalitions. J Pediatr Orthop 2012;32:302; with permission.)

to excision of the coalition.[18,24–32] There is now a general consensus that resection and interposition fat grafting is the treatment of choice for persistently painful middle facet TCCs.[15,16,18,30,32] In 1994, Wilde and colleagues[15] reviewed their results from treating TCCs and found an unsatisfactory result in feet with a CT scan showing a relative coalition area of greater than 50%. In their study, these patients were associated with heel valgus more than 16°, narrowing of the posterior talocalcaneal joint, and impingement of the lateral talar process on the calcaneus. In contrast, patients who had coalitions with a relative area less than 50% were associated with heel valgus less than 16°, normal thickness of the posterior talocalcaneal joint, and absence of impingement of the lateral talar process on the calcaneus. In addition, they described talar beaking as a traction spur as opposed to early degenerative changes found on radiograph, as it did not correlate with clinical outcomes. Talar beaking was present in 33% of feet with a relative coalition size greater than 50% and in 70% of feet with smaller coalitions. In the cases with a relative coalition area greater than 50%, they recommended arthrodesis as opposed to resection.

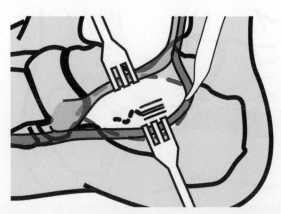

Fig. 6. Resection must go posterior enough to visualize the posterior facet. (*From* Gantsoudes GD, Roocroft JH, Mubarak SJ. Treatment of talocalcaneal coalitions. J Pediatr Orthop 2012;32:303; with permission.)

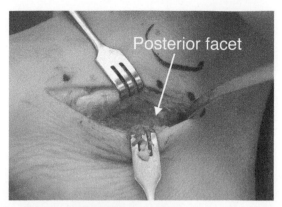

Fig. 7. Intraoperative image showing resection of the posterior facet. (*From* Gantsoudes GD, Roocroft JH, Mubarak SJ. Treatment of talocalcaneal coalitions. J Pediatr Orthop 2012;32:303; with permission.)

In 1998, Luhmann and Schoenecker[16] published their indications and results for symptomatic TCCs. After reviewing their results of 25 coalitions, they recommended that all pediatric and adolescent patients with a symptomatic TCC that failed nonoperative treatment and did not have an arthritic hind foot be treated with a TCC resection as opposed to arthrodesis. They further concluded that patients with TCCs greater than 50% or heel valgus greater than 21° can still have a very satisfactory outcome. However, they did establish that these patients with greater than 21° of hind foot valgus undergo either nonoperative treatment with the use of an orthosis

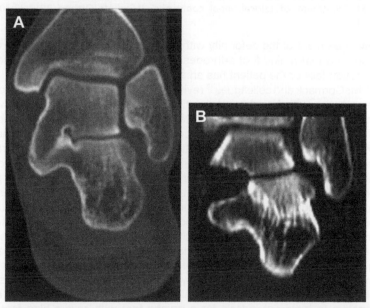

Fig. 8. (*A*) Preoperative axial CT scan. (*B*) Intraoperative CT scan showing complete excision of the lesion. (*From* Kemppainen J, Pennock AT, Mubarak SJ, et al. The use of a portable CT scanner for the intraoperative assessment of talocalcaneal coalition resections. J Pediatr Orthop 2014;34:562; with permission.)

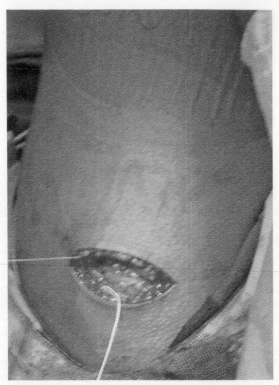

Fig. 9. Fat graft is placed deep to the tendon sheaths. (*From* Gantsoudes GD, Roocroft JH, Mubarak SJ. Treatment of talocalcaneal coalitions. J Pediatr Orthop 2012;32:303; with permission.)

or operative treatment of the deformity with a calcaneal osteotomy or lateral column lengthening, and that a hind foot arthrodesis can be held as a salvage procedure if a TCC resection fails or the patient has an arthritic hindfoot.[16]

In 1997, McCormack and colleagues[31] reviewed 9 symptomatic TCCs that underwent complete resection with fat-graft interposition with a mean duration of follow-up of 11.5 years. In this study, patients had no limitation in range of motion and showed no evidence of degenerative change or joint space narrowing on radiographs. Furthermore, according to the Painful Foot Center questionnaire, 7 feet had an excellent rating, 1 had a fair rating, and 1 a poor rating. Based on these findings, they recommended resection of the middle facet of a persistently symptomatic coalition regardless of percent involvement as long as the patient is without evidence of degenerative changes.

Mosca and colleagues[32] reviewed the short-term to intermediate-term results of 8 patients with 13 symptomatic TCCs that underwent calcaneal lengthening osteotomy for deformity correction with or without coalition resection. In this study, the investigators adhered to recently proposed criteria to determine if a TCC is resectable, including less than 50% the surface area of the posterior facet, less than 16° of hind foot valgus, and with minimal or no narrowing of the posterior facet of the subtalar joint. In this series, they conclude that a calcaneal lengthening osteotomy is a desirable alternative to triple arthrodesis for a painful foot with severe hind foot valgus deformity and an unresectable, solid talocalcaneal tarsal coalition.

Gantsoudes and colleagues[12] from Rady Children's Hospital in San Diego identified 49 feet that underwent TCC resection and fat-graft interposition with at least

12 months of follow-up: 32 had excellent outcomes, 10 had good outcomes, 6 had fair outcomes, and 1 had a poor outcome based on the American Orthopaedic Foot and Ankle Society (AOFAS) Ankle-Hindfoot score. However, when they further categorized patients based on follow-up of 1 to 2 years, 2 to 4 years, or greater than 4 years, the AOFAS scores were not significantly different. This study did not assess preoperative hind foot deformity secondary to the belief that hindfoot valgus and TCC are 2 separate pathologic entities. They concluded that excision to improve range of motion is the best solution to prevent future pathology and to relieve pain, and that correction of preoperative valgus deformity can be necessary as a secondary procedure with similar good results of pain relief.[12] Since the publication of this paper, intraoperative CT scan has become a standard of care in this institution, and the results appear to be improved secondary to more experience and a more thorough TCC resection.

Moraleda and colleagues[33] also investigated the results of the calcaneal lengthening versus the calcaneo-cuboid-cuneiform (Triple C) osteotomies in symptomatic flexible flatfeet. Thirty-three feet underwent a calcaneal lengthening and 30 underwent Triple C osteotomies. Although these patients did not have a TCC, both techniques were found to obtain good clinical and radiographic results at final follow-up when treating symptomatic flexible flatfeet. The calcaneal lengthening osteotomy was found to have better overall correction of the relationship of the navicular to talar head, but was associated with more frequent and more severe complications, including subluxation of the calcaneocuboid joint.[33]

Recently, Mahan and colleagues[34] reviewed patient-reported outcomes of tarsal coalitions treated with surgical excision, and compared the outcomes of TCCs and calcaneonavicular coalitions. They found that 73% of patients with either calcaneonavicular or TC coalition had no activity limitation following surgery, which was correlated with high AOFAS and University of California Los Angeles scores. They also determined that the type of coalition did not impact postoperative outcomes, and concluded that tarsal coalition surgery offers high rates of return to full activity based on patient reports.

SUMMARY

As one can see, there is an abundance of literature to support multiple treatment modalities when approaching TCCs. It is the belief of the authors that TCC and a valgus hindfoot are 2 separate pathologic conditions and are approached as such. First resect the coalition to gain motion and then 6 to 12 months later perform calcaneal, cuboid, and cuneiform osteotomies to correct the flatfoot foot deformity if painful. This was performed in approximately 25% of our patients.

With regard to resection versus arthrodesis for a symptomatic TCC, our preferred treatment is resection with fat-graft interposition in young patients. From previous retrospective reviews and newer literature to support this procedure, we believe it is best to attempt to restore hindfoot motion regardless of the size of coalition. In the older patient with degenerative changes or those who have failed a previous resection, then a triple arthrodesis is a good salvage procedure. However, the literature will suggest only a 20-year life span before ankle arthritis causes this to fail. Therefore, we recommend TCC resection for all pediatric patients and young adults.

REFERENCES

1. Moraleda L, Gantsoudes GD, Mubarak SJ. C Sign: talocalcaneal coalition or flat foot deformity? J Pediatr Orthop 2014;34:814-9.

2. Leonard MA. The inheritance of tarsal coalition and its relationship to spastic flat foot. J Bone Joint Surg Br 1974;56B:520–6.

3. Lateur LM, Van Hoe LR, Van Ghillewe KV, et al. Subtalar coalition: diagnosis with the C sign on lateral radiographs of the ankle. Radiology 1994;193: 847–51.

4. Vincent KA. Tarsal coalition and painful flatfoot. J Am Acad Orthop Surg 1998;6: 274–81.

5. Nalaboff KM, Schweitzer ME. MRI of tarsal coalition: frequency, distribution, and innovative signs. Bull NYU Hosp Jt Dis 2008;66:14–21.

6. Stormont DM, Peterson HA. The relative incidence of tarsal coalition. Clin Orthop Relat Res 1983;181:28–36.

7. Harris RI, Beath T. Etiology of peroneal spastic flat foot. J Bone Joint Surg Br 1948;30:624–34.

8. Vaughan WH, Segal G. Tarsal coalition, with special reference to roentgeno-graphic interpretation. Radiology 1953;60:855–63.

9. Cowell HR. Diagnosis and management of peroneal spastic flatfoot. Instr Course Lect 1975;24:94–103.

10. Cowell HR. Rigid painful flatfoot secondary to tarsal coalition. Clin Orthop Relat Res 1983;177:54–60.

11. Olney BW. Tarsal coalition. In: McCarthy JJ, Drennan JC, editors. Drennan's the Child's foot and ankle. New York: Wolters Kluwer/Lippincott Williams & Wilkins; 2010. p. 160–73.

12. Gantsoudes GD, Roocroft JH, Mubarak SJ. Treatment of talocalcaneal coalitions. J Pediatr Orthop 2012;32:301–7.

13. Moraleda L, Gantsoudes GD, Mubarak SJ. C sign: talocalcaneal coalition of flatfoot deformity? J Pediatr Orthop 2014;34:814–9.

14. Rozansky A, Varley E, Mubarak SJ, et al. A radiologic classification of talocalca-neal coalitions based on 3D reconstruction. J Child Orthop 2010;4:129–35.

15. Wilde PH, Torode IP, Dickens DR, et al. Resection for symptomatic talocalcaneal coalition. J Bone Joint Surg Br 1994;76:797–801.

16. Luhmann SJ, Schoenecker PL. Symptomatic talocalcaneal coalition resection: in-dications and results. J Pediatr Orthop 1998;18:748–54.

17. Khohbin A, Law PW, Caspi L, et al. Long-term functional outcomes of resected tarsal coalitions. Foot Ankle Int 2013;34:1370–5.

18. Olney BW, Asher MA. Excision of symptomatic coalition of the middle facet of the talocalcaneal joint. J Bone Joint Surg Am 1987;69:539–44.

19. Kemppainen J, Pennock AT, Mubarak SJ, et al. The use of a portable CT scanner for the intraoperative assessment of talocalcaneal coalition resections. J Pediatr Orthop 2014;34:559–64.

20. Harris RI. Retrospect—peroneal spastic flat foot (rigid valgus foot). J Bone Joint Surg Am 1965;47:1657–67.

21. Mann RA, Beaman DN, Horton GA. Isolated subtalar arthrodesis. Foot Ankle Int 1998;19:511–9.

22. Mann RA, Baumgarten M. Subtalar fusion for isolated subtalar disorders. Clin Orthop Relat Res 1988;226:260–5.

23. Mosier KM, Asher M. Tarsal coalitions and peroneal spastic flat foot. A review. J Bone Joint Surg Am 1984;66:976–84.

24. Kitaoka HB, Wikenheiser MA, Shaughnessy WJ, et al. Gait abnormalities following resection of talocalcaneal coalition. J Bone Joint Surg Am 1997;79:369–74.

25. Comfort TK, Johnson LO. Resection for symptomatic talocalcaneal coalition. J Pediatr Orthop 1998;18:283–8.

26. Raikin S, Cooperman DR, Thompson GH. Interposition of the split flexor hallucis longus tendon after resection of a coalition of the middle facet of the talocalcaneal joint. J Bone Joint Surg Am 1999;81:11–9.
27. Kumar SJ, Guille JT, Lee MS, et al. Osseous and non-osseous coalition of the middle facet of the talocalcaneal joint. J Bone Joint Surg Am 1992;74:529–35.
28. Saxena A, Erickson S. Tarsal coalitions. Activity levels with and without surgery. J Am Podiatr Med Assoc 2003;93:259–63.
29. Dutoit M. Talocalcaneal bar resection. J Foot Ankle Surg 1998;37:199–203.
30. Scranton PE Jr. Treatment of symptomatic talocalcaneal coalition. J Bone Joint Surg Am 1987;69:533–9.
31. McCormack TJ, Olney B, Asher M. Talocalcaneal coalition resection: a 10-year follow-up. J Pediatr Orthop 1997;17:13–5.
32. Mosca VS, Bevan WP. Talocalcaneal tarsal coalitions and the calcaneal lengthening osteotomy: the role of deformity correction. J Bone Joint Surg Am 2012; 94:1584–94.
33. Moraleda L, Salcedo M, Bastrom TP, et al. Comparison of the calcaneo-cuboid-cuneiform osteotomies and the calcaneal lengthening osteotomy in the surgical treatment of symptomatic flexible flatfoot. J Pediatr Orthop 2012;32:821–9.
34. Mahan ST, Spencer SA, Kasser JR, et al. Patient-reported outcomes of tarsal coalitions treated with surgical excision. J Pediatr Orthop 2015;35(6):683–8.

Painful Flexible Flatfoot

Abdel Majid Sheikh Taha, MD, David S. Feldman, MD*

KEYWORDS

- Flexible flatfoot • Pes planovalgus • Pes equinovalgus • Treatment • Pain

KEY POINTS

- Flexible flatfoot (FFF) has 2 subtypes: pes planovalgus and pes equinovalgus.
- Most FFF patients are asymptomatic and only those that become symptomatic require treatment.
- Conservative treatment remains the mainstay in FFF and it is usually in the form of arch support orthotics and exercises.
- Surgical intervention, using arthrodesis or nonarthrodesis procedures, is warranted when conservative treatment fails.
- Nonarthrodesis procedures are preferred and arthrodesis procedures are the last resort when all other treatments fail.

BACKGROUND

No study in the literature adequately defines flatfoot in terms of measurable radiographic or clinical values.[1] The absence of the medial arch, the hindfoot valgus, and the relative forefoot to midfoot supination define this entity. A flatfoot is called "flexible" when forefoot supination and dorsiflexion of the hallux in a weight-bearing position restores the arch, a positive Jack's test (**Fig. 1**).[2] It is the most common form of flatfoot. We distinguish 2 subtypes of flexible flatfoot (FFF): pes planovalgus and pes equinovalgus. The hallmark between the subtypes is the tightness of the heel cord. As the name implies, the heel cord is tight in the equinovalgus form. Clinically, bringing the hindfoot into neutral allows the differentiation between the two. Harris and Beath[3] were the first to describe pes equinovalgus using the term "hypermobile flatfoot" in a cohort of Canadian soldiers. Characteristics of the hypermobile flatfoot are persistent since childhood, corrects when unloaded from weight bearing, associated with a short tendoachilles, and has abnormal relationships of the tarsal bones. The incidence of symptoms is higher in this group of patients.[3]

The authors have nothing to disclose.
Department of Orthopaedic Surgery, New York University Langone Medical Center, New York, NY 10003, USA
* Corresponding author.
E-mail address: David.Feldman@nyumc.org

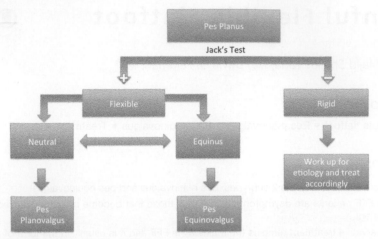

Fig. 1. Diagnosis algorithm for flatfoot.

DEVELOPMENT AND RISK FACTORS

Reports regarding the true incidence of FFF vary. Harris and Beath had the largest cohort of FFF looking into the incidence in 3619 Canadian soldiers.[1,3–5] In their study, these authors reported a 20% incidence of FFF. The many factors associated with flatfoot include age, gender, ethnicity, and shoe wearing. Early in life, flatfoot is a normal stage of development. The medial arch develops through the normal process of growing.[6–9] Vanderwilde and colleagues[8] studied a population of normal children in Columbia in the first 5 years of life. They concluded that young children are flatfooted and the arch develops as they grow beyond 5 years of age. Another study conducted in Austria showed similar results and exhibited a reduction of flatfoot in more than 50% of the children between the ages of 3 and 6 years.[10] Other authors looked into the effect of shoe wearing and found that FFF was more prevalent in the shod versus the unshod children.[11,12] Flatfoot occurs more frequently among obese school children.[13–17] Ethnicity can also play a role, with a higher incidence of flatfoot in African-Americans compared with Caucasians.[18–20]

The several theories defining the etiology of FFF depend on the anatomy of the foot and the surrounding musculature. The earliest theories focused on muscle imbalance and weakness around the foot as the primary causes of flatfootedness.[21] Later, the bony anatomy and the ligamentous laxity of the midfoot joints were proposed as the main factor.[22–24] Harris and Beath[3] distinguished between the passive and the active support of the foot. The passive support is the bony and the ligamentous structures of the foot. The active support is the muscular envelope that includes muscles belonging to the foot alone and others that insert in the foot but originate in the leg. The passive support is the primary arch support and the active support comes into play when the passive support fails. Basmajian and Stecko[24] studied the muscle electrophysiology while applying different loads to the foot. They concluded that the bony and ligamentous structures are the primary restraints of the arch and that the muscles come into play with excessive loads.[25] These muscles play a principal, active role in the stabilization of the foot during propulsion.[25]

PATHOPHYSIOLOGY

To understand the pathophysiology of the flatfoot and the principles of treatment, one must be aware of the importance of the subtalar and the midtarsal anatomy.[26] The subtalar joint is composed of the anterior and the posterior talocalcaneal articulation. The anterior articulation is between the biconcave facet of the calcaneus and the anterior convex surface of the talar head and posterior convex surface of the navicular. The posterior articulation is between the posterior convex facet of the calcaneus and the concave talar facet. The calcaneus supports the talar head and neck, which in turn supports the navicular. The interosseous talocalcaneal ligament supports the subtalar joint. This ligament blends with the talocalcaneonavicular joint anteriorly and the subtalar joint capsule posteriorly. The motion that results around the axis of rotation of the subtalar joint is "out and up" or "in and down" (**Fig. 2**).

The midtarsal joints are the talonavicular and the calcaneocuboid joints. The former is a ball-and-socket and the latter is a trochlear joint. These joints allow for minimal motion: dorsiflexion, plantar flexion, and forefoot rotation on the hindfoot. Knowledge of these relationships allows a better understanding of the effect of the various interventions available for managing flatfeet.

The subtalar and the midtarsal joints act as the mechanical connection between the foot and the tibia.[26] Loads from the body and the lower limb are transmitted through these joints to the foot. Motion through these joints orchestrates the ongoing transformation of the foot from a supple configuration to accommodate the ground during weight bearing to a rigid one to assist in push-off toward the end of stance. The foot deformity in FFF has 3 components: forefoot hyperabduction, forefoot supination, and hindfoot valgus. This deformity renders the foot supple at all times thus loosing its contribution to push-off.[27,28] It is not only a static malalignment of the foot and ankle, but also a functional change of the lower limb dynamics.[29]

Flatfoot has been reported as a risk of overuse injuries in people with high demand, including athletes and soldiers.[30] Kaufman and colleagues[31] found that the presence of flatfoot is a risk factor for overuse injuries particularly stress fractures. These findings contradicted those of Cowan and Giladi that pes planus was protective against the aforementioned injuries.[30,32]

PRESENTATION AND PHYSICAL EXAMINATION

Most patients with flatfoot who come for medical attention do so regarding cosmesis and shoe wear, but most often do not complain of pain. The symptomatic patients primarily seek treatment owing to pain and at times, a decrease in function. Flatfoot pain is usually induced by strenuous activity and relieved by rest. This pattern applies to both the flexible as well as the rigid types. Pain may be located over the medial aspect of the heel, the sinus tarsi, the distal fibula, and the medial aspect of the midfoot. Other diagnoses should be sought if this pain occurs during the night and awakens the patient from sleep.

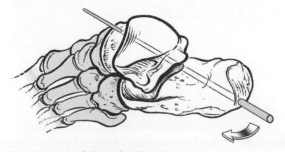

Fig. 2. Axis of rotation (*arrow*) of the subtalar joint.

The physical examination of the child or adolescent with a FFF starts with barefoot gait observation. Depending on the severity of the flatfoot, the gait demonstrates varying degrees of forefoot abduction. Forefoot abduction is also the reason behind the too-many-toes sign noted by the examiner when inspecting the child's feet from behind (**Fig. 3**). The absence of the medial arch is also noted (**Fig. 4**) and is usually restored when the child is asked to stand on tiptoe (**Fig. 5**) or when the hallux is brought into dorsiflexion in the weight-bearing foot, a positive Jack's test (**Fig. 6**). Shoes are examined for signs of medial wear. The rest of the examination is carried out with the patient seated. The medial aspect of the foot is inspected for hypertrophied skin and callosities. The hindfoot is locked in neutral and dorsiflexion is performed looking for a tight Achilles tendon, thus differentiating between the equinovalgus and the planovalgus subtypes of FFF (**Fig. 7**). Examining the child for any signs of joint laxity and hypermobility should be a part of the evaluation.

Evaluation of rotational deformity is essential because, when present, it can mask or exacerbate the appearance of the flatfoot deformity. This examination includes assessing the femoral version and the tibial torsion. The femoral version is assessed clinically by examining hip rotation and performing the trochanteric prominence angle test. The thigh–foot angle reflects the direction and amount of tibial torsion.[33–35] This test is best performed with the patient lying in the prone position. Imaging version studies are warranted when signs of rotational malalignment are found.

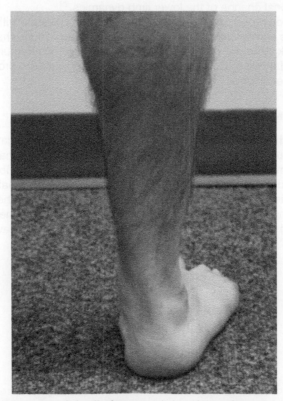

Fig. 3. Posterior inspection of the flatfoot reveals hindfoot valgus and the too-many-toes sign secondary to forefoot hyperabduction.

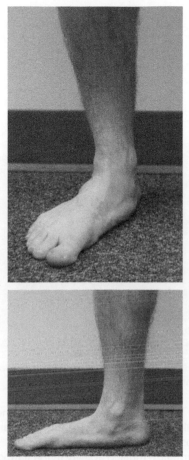

Fig. 4. Anterior and side views of the weight-bearing flatfoot demonstrate the absence of the medial arch and the forefoot hyperabduction.

Radiographs are usually reserved for symptomatic patients with flatfoot. The radiographic evaluation consists of a dorsoplantar and a lateral projection of the foot. A Harris view and sometimes a computed tomography or MRI or both are added to the evaluation in the case of rigid flatfoot to look for a tarsal coalition, but this evaluation is not within the scope of this review. On the lateral view, the plantar sag of the talonavicular joint is appreciated. The angles that are usually measured are the talus–first metatarsal angle, talocalcaneal angle, and the calcaneal pitch (**Fig. 8**).[36] These angles are used to follow the amount of correction achieved by an intervention, whether operative or nonoperative. On the dorsoplantar view, the talus–first metatarsal angle, the talonavicular coverage angle, and the talonavicular percent uncoverage are appreciated (**Fig. 9**).[36,37]

MANAGEMENT

The management of flatfoot depends on the presence or absence of symptoms and the duration of these symptoms. The management of the symptomatic patient usually starts with conservative intervention, which includes the use of orthotics and physical

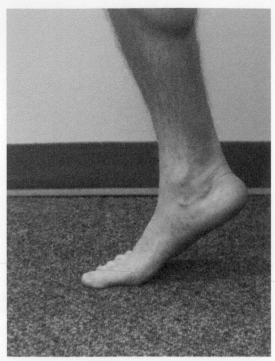

Fig. 5. Tiptoeing puts the hallux in dorsiflexion and the hindfoot in neutral, restoring the medial arch in a flexible flatfoot.

therapy. Physical therapy may include exercises to strengthen the arch as well as to teach a program for Achilles stretching. The literature contains conflicting reports on the efficacy of using orthoses for the treatment of flatfoot.[38–43] Customized and modified foot orthoses may normalize muscle activity in the flatfoot.[41] The Helfet heel seat shoe orthoses was introduced in 1956 for the treatment of the FFF[44] followed by the University of California Biomechanical Laboratory shoe insert in 1976.[45] The aim of using foot orthoses is to put the foot in a biomechanically better position to function.[39] Their mode of action is believed to rely on limiting subtalar motion, decreasing hindfoot eversion, and fixing the hindfoot in neutral, thus restoring the medial arch. Banwell and colleagues[38] performed a systematic review of the use of foot orthoses in FFF.

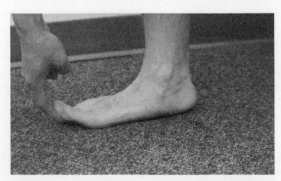

Fig. 6. Dorsiflexion of the hallux restores the medial arch in a flexible flatfoot (Jack's test).

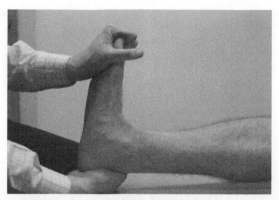

Fig. 7. Holding the hindfoot in neutral and applying dorsiflexion to the foot distinguish pes planovalgus from pes equinovalgus.

Despite the moderate evidence that the use of foot orthoses may improve physical function, the evidence supporting their effectiveness in reducing pain and decreasing hindfoot eversion remains low.[38] Hard foot orthoses should be avoided in rigid flatfoot or the pes equinovalgus form in which exacerbation rather than relief of symptoms occurs. Soft gel pads should be used instead. Concomitantly, a heel cord stretching protocol should be initiated for an associated tight Achilles tendon. Patients who do not respond to conservative treatment are indicated for a surgical intervention. There is no defined cutoff for the duration of conservative treatment. The decision to transition to a surgical intervention should rely on the persistence and the lack of improvement in symptoms rather than cosmesis of the foot, which is usually the primary concern of the child's parents or caregivers. Inability to wear shoes comfortably may be another reason to move forward with surgical intervention.

PROCEDURES

The many procedures that have been described for the treatment of flatfoot can be divided into 2 categories: arthrodesis and nonarthrodesis procedures. Nonarthrodesis procedures have become the mainstay of surgical intervention. These techniques include reconstructive foot surgery and arthroereisis.

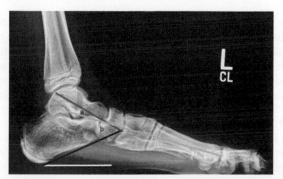

Fig. 8. Lateral radiograph showing the different radiographic measurements: the lateral talus–first metatarsal angle *a* (*red line* and *green line*), the talocalcaneal angle *b* (*red line* and *black line*), and the calcaneal pitch angle *c* (*black line* and *white line*).

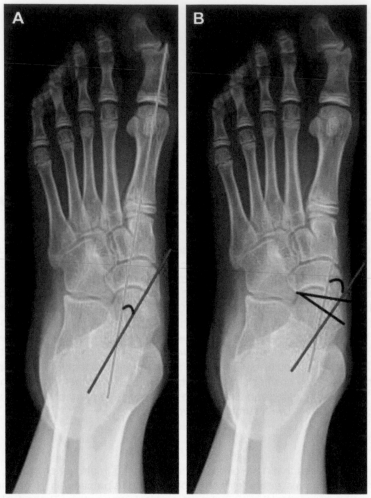

Fig. 9. Dorsoplantar radiograph showing (*A*) the talus–first MT angle and (*B*) the talonavic-ular coverage angle.

Reconstructive surgery includes soft tissue procedures used in conjunction with the realignment osteotomies. Soft tissue procedures alone, such as peroneus brevis with achilles lengthening, are ineffective and rarely indicated. The ultimate goal is to realign the hindfoot and correct the forefoot hyperabduction to restore a normal relationship of the foot to the weight-bearing line. The soft tissue procedures include lengthening of the peroneus brevis, talonavicular capsulorraphy, and posterior tibial advancement.[46–49] An Achilles tendon lengthening procedure is added depending on the status of the heel cord. Various bony procedures have been described. The difference is the number, location, and type of the osteotomies used. Anderson and Fowler[49] described an anterior calcaneal osteotomy for the treatment of FFF. These authors performed the osteotomy 4 mm proximal to the calcaneocuboid joint. The most popular and cited procedure in the literature is the lateral column length-ening osteotomy described by Evans[50] and later modified by Mosca.[46] Both osteot-omies are done 1.5 cm proximal to the calcaneocuboid joint. Mosca's modifications of the Evan's procedure include a cosmetically more acceptable incision, an oblique osteotomy directed from proximal–lateral to distal–medial when compared with the classic straight osteotomy, the use of internal fixation, and the addition of the release of the abductor digiti minimi aponeurosis and the lateral plantar fascia, as well as the lengthening of the peronei as needed based on the intraoperative findings.[46,50] Rathjen and Mubarak[47] described an alternative technique that involved osteotomies of the calcaneus, cuboid and cuneiform. This was later referred to as the triple C osteotomy by Bouchard and Mosca.[48] A posterior translational osteotomy of the os calcis is another option if heel valgus needs to be addressed alone.[47,48,51]

Arthroereisis involves inserting a peg in the sinus tarsi to limit hindfoot eversion. The principle behind this procedure is blocking the lineal displacement of the talus during gait, which in turn stops the other components of pronation, namely calcaneal eversion, talar adduction, and plantar flexion.[52] Indications and contraindications for this procedure have not been delineated clearly. Persistent pain, overcorrection, and undercorrection have been reported.[53]

Arthrodesing procedures vary from selective mid-tarsal to triple arthrodesis. The most cited midtarsal procedure is the naviculocuneiform fusion.[54–56] Hoke described the navicular to medial and middle cuneiforms arthrodeses in 1931.[54,56,57] This procedure was a purely bony procedure and he relied on a plaster cast to achieve and maintain his correction.[54] Miller's procedure, on the other hand, fuses 2 joints: the navicular–medial cuneiform and cuneiform–first metatarsal joints. The advancement of the calcaneonavicular ligament and the posterior tibialis tendon is included in the procedure.[55,58] Duncan and Lovell[56] described a modified Hoke–Miller procedure that involves the fusion of the naviculo-medial cuneiform joint and the advancement of a subperiosteal flap to the plantar fascia to tension the latter to hold the corrected arch. Selective fusions have demonstrated good short-term results.[54,58,59] They all share the lack of long-term detailed follow-up.[56] Later, triple arthrodesis was used in the treatment of FFF. Long-term follow-up studies revealed good to excellent results in two-thirds of patients.[26] Arthrodesis procedures lead to arthritis in adjacent joints, although this finding was asymptomatic in some reports.[26,60] Procedures that combine reconstruction to realign the foot with triple arthrodesis are also described to treat FFF. Frost and colleagues[61] reported good results combining triple arthrodesis with lateral column lengthening of the calcaneus. Arthrodesis procedures should be kept as a last resort when other reconstructive options fail or when arthritis of the joints is symptomatic.

REFERENCES

1. Mosca VS. Flexible flatfoot and skewfoot. Instr Course Lect 1996;45:347–54.
2. Jack EA. Naviculo-cuneiform fusion in the treatment of flat foot. J Bone Joint Surg Br 1953;35-B(1):75–82.
3. Harris R, Beath T. Hypermobile flat foot with short TA. J Bone Joint Surg Am 1948; 30A(1):116–40.
4. Halabchi F, Mazaheri R, Mirshahi M, et al. Pediatric flatfoot: an algorithmic clinical approach. Iran J Pediatr 2013;23(3):247–60.
5. Tenenbaum S, Hershkovich O, Gordon B, et al. Flexible pes planus in adolescents: body mass index, body height, and gender–an epidemiological study. Foot Ankle Int 2013;34(6):811–7.
6. Gould N, Moreland M, Alvarez R. Development of the child's arch. Foot Ankle 1989;9(5):241–5.

7. Staheli LT, Chew DE, Corbett M. The longitudinal arch: a survey of eight hundred and eighty-two feet in normal children and adults. J Bone Joint Surg Am 1987; 69(3):426–8.
8. Vanderwilde R, Staheli LT, Chew DE, et al. Measurements on radiographs of the foot in normal infants and children. J Bone Joint Surg Am 1988;70(3):407–15.
9. Onodera AN, Sacco IC, Morioka EH, et al. What is the best method for child longitudinal plantar arch assessment and when does arch maturation occur? Foot (Edinb) 2008;18(3):142–9.
10. Pfeiffer M, Kotz R, Ledl T, et al. Prevalence of flat foot in preschool-aged children. Pediatrics 2006;118(2):634–9.
11. Sim-Fook L, Hodgson AR. A comparison of foot forms among the non-shoe and the shoe-wearing Chinese population. J Bone Joint Surg Am 1958;40-A(5): 1058–62.
12. Rao UB, Joseph B. The influence of footwear on the prevalence of flat foot. A survey of 2300 children. J Bone Joint Surg Br 1992;74(4):525–7.
13. Shultz SP, Anner J, Hills AP. Paediatric obesity, physical activity and the musculoskeletal system. Obes Rev 2009;10(5):576–82.
14. Dowling AM, Steele JR, Baur LA. Does obesity influence foot structure and plantar pressure patterns in prepubescent children? Int J Obes Relat Metab Disord 2001;25(6):845–52.
15. Riddiford-Harland DL, Steele JR, Storlien LH. Does obesity influence foot structure in prepubescent children? Int J Obes Relat Metab Disord 2000;24(5):541–4.
16. Hills AP, Hennig EM, Byrne NM, et al. The biomechanics of adiposity–structural and functional limitations of obesity and implications for movement. Obes Rev 2002;3(1):35–43.
17. Bordin D, De Giorgi G, Mazzocco G, et al. Flat and cavus foot, indexes of obesity and overweight in a population of primary-school children. Minerva Pediatr 2001; 53(1):7–13.
18. Golightly YM, Hannan MT, Dufour AB, et al. Racial differences in foot disorders and foot type. Arthritis Care Res (Hoboken) 2012;64(11):1756–9.
19. Castro-Aragon O, Vallurupalli S, Warner M, et al. Ethnic radiographic foot differences. Foot Ankle Int 2009;30(1):57–61.
20. Stewart SF. Human gait and the human foot: an ethnological study of flatfoot. I. Clin Orthop Relat Res 1970;70:111–23.
21. Keith A. The history of the human foot and its weight bearing on orthopaedic practice. J Bone Joint Surg Am 1929;11(1):10–32.
22. Morton DJ, Fuller DD. Human locomotion and body form. A study of gravity and man. Baltimore (MD): The Williams and Wilkins Co; 1952. p. 74.
23. Morton DJ. The human foot. New York: Columbia University Press; 1935. p. 119.
24. Basmajian JV, Stecko G. The role of muscles in arch support of the foot. J Bone Joint Surg Am 1963;45:1184–90.
25. Mann R, Inman VT. Phasic activity of intrinsic muscles of the foot. J Bone Joint Surg Am 1964;46:469–81.
26. Adelaar RS, Dannelly EA, Meunier PA, et al. A long term study of triple arthrodesis in children. Orthop Clin North Am 1976;7(4):895–908.
27. Bordelon RL. Hypermobile flatfoot in children. Comprehension, evaluation, and treatment. Clin Orthop Relat Res 1983;(181):7–14.
28. Morris JM. Biomechanics of the foot and ankle. Clin Orthop Relat Res 1977;(122): 10–7.
29. Lin CJ, Lai KA, Kuan TS, et al. Correlating factors and clinical significance of flexible flatfoot in preschool children. J Pediatr Orthop 2001;21(3):378–82.

30. Cowan DN, Jones BH, Robinson JR. Foot morphologic characteristics and risk of exercise-related injury. Arch Fam Med 1993;2(7):773–7.
31. Kaufman KR, Brodine SK, Shaffer RA, et al. The effect of foot structure and range of motion on musculoskeletal overuse injuries. Am J Sports Med 1999;27(5): 585–93.
32. Giladi M, Milgrom C, Stein M. The low arch, a protective factor in stress fractures: a prospective study of 295 military recruits. Orthop Rev 1985;14:709–12.
33. Chung CY, Lee KM, Park MS, et al. Validity and reliability of measuring femoral anteversion and neck-shaft angle in patients with cerebral palsy. J Bone Joint Surg Am 2010;92(5):1195–205.
34. Staheli LT, Corbett M, Wyss C, et al. Lower-extremity rotational problems in children. Normal values to guide management. J Bone Joint Surg Am 1985;67(1):39–47.
35. Staheli LT. Rotational problems of the lower extremities. Orthop Clin North Am 1987;18(4):503–12.
36. Davids JR, Gibson TW, Pugh LI. Quantitative segmental analysis of weight-bearing radiographs of the foot and ankle for children: normal alignment. J Pediatr Orthop 2005;25(6):769–76.
37. Steel MW, Johnson KA, Dewitz MA, et al. Radiographic measurements of the normal adult foot. Foot Ankle 1980;1(3):151–8.
38. Banwell HA, Mackintosh S, Thewlis D. Foot orthoses for adults with flexible pes planus: a systematic review. J Foot Ankle Res 2014;7(1):23.
39. Bleck EE, Berzins UJ. Conservative management of pes valgus with plantar flexed talus, flexible. Clin Orthop Relat Res 1977;(122):85–94.
40. Penneau K, Lutter LD, Winter RD. Pes planus: radiographic changes with foot orthoses and shoes. Foot Ankle 1982;2(5):299–303.
41. Murley GS, Landorf KB, Menz HB. Do foot orthoses change lower limb muscle activity in flat-arched feet towards a pattern observed in normal-arched feet? Clin Biomech (Bristol, Avon) 2010;25(7):728–36.
42. Zifchock RA, Davis I. A comparison of semi-custom and custom foot orthotic devices in high- and low-arched individuals during walking. Clin Biomech (Bristol, Avon) 2008;23(10):1287–93.
43. Wenger DR, Mauldin D, Speck G, et al. Corrective shoes and inserts as treatment for flexible flatfoot in infants and children. J Bone Joint Surg Am 1989;71(6): 800–10.
44. Helfet AJ. A new way of treating flat feet in children. Lancet 1956;270(6911): 262–4.
45. Henderson WH, Campbell JW. UCBL shoe insert: casting and fabrication. San Francisco: The Biomechanics Laboratory, University of California at San Francisco and Berkeley; 1967. Technical Report 53.
46. Mosca VS. Calcaneal lengthening for valgus deformity of the hindfoot. Results in children who had severe, symptomatic flatfoot and skewfoot. J Bone Joint Surg Am 1995;77(4):500–12.
47. Rathjen KE, Mubarak SJ. Calcaneal-cuboid-cuneiform osteotomy for the correction of valgus foot deformities in children. J Pediatr Orthop 1998;18(6):775–82.
48. Bouchard M, Mosca VS. Flatfoot deformity in children and adolescents: surgical indications and management. J Am Acad Orthop Surg 2014;22(10):623–32.
49. Anderson AF, Fowler SB. Anterior calcaneal osteotomy for symptomatic juvenile pes planus. Foot Ankle 1984;4(5):274–83.
50. Evans D. Calcaneovalgus deformity. J Bone Joint Surg Br 1975;57:270–8.
51. Dwyer FC. Osteotomy of the calcaneum for pes cavus. J Bone Joint Surg Br 1959;41-B(1):80–6.

52. Smith SD, Millar EA. Arthrorisis by means of a subtalar polyethylene peg implant for correction of hindfoot pronation in children. Clin Orthop Relat Res 1983;(181): 15–23.
53. Grady JF, Dinnon MW. Subtalar arthroereisis in the neurologically normal child. Clin Podiatr Med Surg 2000;17(3):443–57, vi.
54. Hoke M. An operation for the correction of extremely relaxed flatfeet. J Bone Joint Surg 1931;13:773–83.
55. Miller OL. A plastic flatfoot operation. J Bone Joint Surg 1927;9:84–91.
56. Duncan JW, Lovell WW. Modified Hoke-Miller flatfoot procedure. Clin Orthop Relat Res 1983;(181):24–7.
57. Butte FL. Navicular-cuneiform arthrodesis for flatfoot. J Bone Joint Surg 1937;19: 496–502.
58. Fraser RK, Menelaus MB, Williams PF, et al. The Miller procedure for mobile flat feet. J Bone Joint Surg Br 1995;77(3):396–9.
59. Crego CH Jr, Ford LT. An end-result of various operative procedures for correcting flat feet in children. J Bone Joint Surg Am 1952;34-A(1):183–95.
60. Ebalard M, Le Henaff G, Sigonney G, et al. Risk of osteoarthritis secondary to partial or total arthrodesis of the subtalar and midtarsal joints after a minimum follow-up of 10 years. Orthop Traumatol Surg Res 2014;100(4):S231–7.
61. Frost NL, Grassbaugh JA, Baird G, et al. Triple arthrodesis with lateral column lengthening for the treatment of planovalgus deformity. J Pediatr Orthop 2011; 31(7):773–82.

Pediatric Ankle Fractures
Concepts and Treatment Principles

Alvin W. Su, MD, PhD[a,b], A. Noelle Larson, MD[a,*]

KEYWORDS

- Ankle fracture • Salter-Harris • Growth plate injury • Physis • Transitional fracture
- Pediatric sports injury • Ankle trauma • Leg length discrepancy

KEY POINTS

- Pediatric ankle fractures account for 15% of all physeal injuries.
- The Salter-Harris classification is the most widely adopted system.
- Salter-Harris type III and IV fractures more frequently require operative treatment and may result in growth arrest.
- Local soft tissue swelling and inability to bear weight should prompt radiographs to assess for fracture.
- Tillaux and triplane injuries are specific fracture patterns that occur as the physis closes, may be missed on plain radiographs, and frequently require surgical management to restore congruency of the articular surface.

SCOPE OF REVIEW

The present review discusses pediatric ankle fractures, defined as tibia and fibula fractures distal to the metaphysis in patients with open physes. Most of these fractures are caused by sports injuries or low-energy trauma.[1] The pediatric ankle with open physes and incomplete ossification presents distinct mechanical and biological properties compared to the skeletally mature ankle. Thus, children have unique ankle fracture patterns and require specific treatment to preserve and monitor the physis.

EPIDEMIOLOGY

Ankle fractures represent around 5% of all fractures, 15–20% of all physeal injuries in children, and are the most common physeal injury in the lower extremity.[2–5] Ankle

Institutional Review Board approval was obtained for this study.
The authors have nothing to disclose.
[a] Department of Orthopedic Surgery, Mayo Clinic, 200 1st Street Southwest, Rochester, MN 55905, USA; [b] School of Medicine, National Yang-Ming University, No. 155, Section 2, Linong Street, Beitou, Taipei, Taiwan
* Corresponding author.
E-mail address: larson.noelle@mayo.edu

fractures also occur in adolescents and more frequently require surgical management than distal radius fractures and other fractures. There is a higher incidence of ankle fractures in children with increased body mass index.[6,7] Basketball, soccer, football, and scooters are the most common activities associated with ankle fractures.[8–11]

PEDIATRIC ANKLE ANATOMY

Of all physeal injuries, fractures of the distal tibial physis have among the highest rates of complications, including premature physeal arrest, bar formation, angular deformity, and articular incongruity.[12,13] The physis contains 4 zones, from the epiphysis to the metaphysis, with decreasing mechanical strength caused by decreasing matrix-cell ratio: the reserve zone, the proliferative zone, the hypertrophic zone, and the provisional calcification zone. Fracture typically occurs through the hypertrophic zone, which has the largest cells and less extracellular matrix than the other zones. For most fractures, this in turn preserves the reserve zone, which is located on the epiphyseal side of the fracture and contains the progenitor cells for physeal growth.[14,15] Fractures that cross the physis into the epiphysis (Salter-Harris [SH] types III and IV), however, may damage the reserve zone and, thus, are at higher risk of causing physeal growth disturbance.

The distal tibial physis provides 40% of the growth of the tibia and 17% of lower extremity growth, with 3 to 4 mm of growth per year in childhood. Distal tibial growth occurs proportionately to the proximal tibia in young patients; but in adolescents, the proximal tibia growth becomes more rapid and distal tibial growth tapers off.[16] Thus, injury to the physis at a young age can result in significant leg length discrepancy. The distal tibial ossification center appears around 6 months of age and the distal fibula around 1 to 3 years of age. Distal tibial and fibular physeal closure occurs around 12 to 17 years of age in girls and 15 to 20 years of age in boys.[17,18] In contrast to other physes, tibial physeal closure occurs slowly and eccentrically, beginning around the Poland hump, and then anteromedially, posterolaterally, and finally anterolaterally. This pattern of closure explains the specific tibial physeal fracture patterns seen in adolescent triplane and Tillaux fractures. Physeal arrest is generally not a concern for triplane and Tillaux fractures, because the physis is already closing in these fracture patterns. Abundant blood supply is provided to the distal tibial physis, so posttraumatic avascular necrosis of the plafond is very rare.

The distal fibula is contained in a groove on the lateral distal tibia and has significant ligamentous constraint with the anterior and posterior tibiofibular and calcaneofibular ligaments. Ligamentous structures in children are quite robust, whereas the physis is biomechanically vulnerable to shear and rotational forces. Thus, the same injury mechanism that may result in an ankle sprain in adults can present with physeal or avulsion fractures in children. The distal fibula physis becomes undulating during childhood, which does provide it with additional stability.[18] The distal fibula frequently has a secondary center of ossification that can mimic an avulsion fracture on radiograph. The medial os subtibiale is more prevalent than the lateral os subfibulare.[19,20] Clinical examination findings may be used to distinguish a nondisplaced avulsion fracture from an ossification center.

Growth of the fibula is evenly distributed between the proximal and distal fibular physis in childhood, although the proximal fibular growth becomes predominant in adolescents.[21] Isolated physeal arrest of the fibula is rare but can lead to ankle valgus and an external foot progression angle.

PATIENT EVALUATION AND DIAGNOSIS

History

Patients frequently present following a twisting injury to the ankle. It is important to distinguish an ankle fracture from an ankle sprain. Hallmark findings include inability to bear weight, bony tenderness, swelling, or deformity.

Physical Examination

The skin should be evaluated for open wounds, ecchymoses, or abrasions. Edema and discoloration may develop over the first 24 to 48 hours after injury. Neurovascular status should be assessed, including a sensory examination, palpation of pulses, and testing of capillary refill. Then a focused examination should evaluate the site of maximal tenderness, specifically examining the distal tibial and fibular physes, medial and lateral malleoli, tibial and fibula shafts, the base of the fifth metatarsal, and the peroneal tendons. A fifth metatarsal fracture or peroneal tendon subluxation may mimic an ankle fracture. Ligamentous structures should also be evaluated, including anterior and posterior talofibular ligaments, calcaneofibular ligaments, and anterior tibiofibular ligament. Maximal tenderness over the ligaments distal to the malleoli may indicate sprain rather than fracture. If the patients' condition will tolerate, a squeeze test can be performed proximally and a stress test of the medial ligamentous complex with passive flexion and external rotation of the foot to assess for a ligamentous or syndesmotic injury.

Atypical Fractures

The treating physician should always assess for atypical presentations, such as absent or inadequate trauma history, antecedent pain, or constitutional symptoms. Small children are particularly at risk for misdiagnosis, as they may not be able to recount an episode of trauma and can develop hematogenous osteomyelitis with no associated risk factors. Less common causes of atypical fractures include nonaccidental trauma or leukemia. Radiographs should always be evaluated for a lytic lesion or periosteal reaction adjacent to the fracture site. In addition, a history that does not match the presenting injury pattern should alert the physician of possible child abuse. Nearly half of the child abuse cases present with solitary fracture alone.[22]

Radiographs

Ankle radiographs with 3 views should be used to selectively evaluate for fracture in patients with ankle injuries. The Ottawa Rules (bony tenderness along the malleoli, inability to bear weight) were developed for adults to help determine when radiographs are necessary[23] and have been validated for children[24,25] but have been criticized for having a high false-negative rate in adults.[26,27] The Low Risk Ankle Rule has also been developed specifically for children to determine when a radiograph is needed and has been shown to reduce the number of radiographs and result in cost savings in the emergency department.[28] Low-risk ankle injuries are defined as sprains, nondisplaced SH-I and SH-II fractures, and avulsion fractures of the distal fibula. Radiographs are not required if there is only tenderness of the distal fibula or adjacent lateral ligaments.[29]

Radiographic images should be evaluated for physeal widening, which may indicate a SH-I fracture. The plafond and mortise should be carefully examined for evidence of an intra-articular fracture pattern, such as a Tillaux or triplane fracture, as these findings can be quite subtle. A SH-II fracture of the fibula may only be visible on the lateral view and will be superimposed on the image of the lateral tibia. If displaced, this may result in a growth arrest.

If radiographs are suspicious for an intra-articular fracture pattern, computed to-mography (CT) imaging may be obtained to evaluate articular congruity, assess the need for surgical management, and assist in preoperative planning. This imaging is most commonly indicated for Tillaux and triplane fractures, as most SH fractures can be assessed and treated without axial imaging. After viewing CT imaging, sur-geons more frequently recommend surgical treatment of Tillaux and triplane fractures because of the significant intra-articular step-offs that are difficult to appreciate on plain films.[30] An MRI may provide similar information but has increased costs and at most centers is not as readily obtained as CT. Several reports show MRI specifically does not change the treatment plan for acute pediatric ankle fractures.[31,32] It may, however, provide information for surgical planning, characterize suspected osteo-chondral injury, or rule out underlying tumor or infection.

Routine ankle stress views are not recommended for most pediatric ankle fractures. However, for adult ankle fracture equivalents (supination external rotation pattern), a gravity stress view may be a useful tool to assess whether surgical management is indi-cated and whether weight bearing can be initiated immediately.[33,34] Gravity stress views are well tolerated and less painful than the traditional manual stress radiographs.[33,34]

FRACTURE CLASSIFICATION

The SH classification is the most widely recognized system to describe physeal injuries.[13,35] This system is easy to apply, has good interobserver and intraobserver reliability, and provides valuable prognostic information regarding growth arrest and subsequent complications.

The Dias-Tachdjian classification categorizes pediatric ankle fractures based on the applied traumatic force to the foot and the position of the foot when it sustains such force. If the pattern is recognized correctly, this system can potentially help fracture reduction by reversing the applied force. However, the low interobserver reliability and its complex nature render the system less popular. The Peterson classification has also been described.[36,37]

Salter-Harris Classification

The most common physeal ankle fracture is the SH type II (SH-II), which account for 32% to 40% of pediatric distal tibial fractures, then followed by SH-III (25%), SH-IV (up to 25%), SH-I (3%–15%), and SH-V (less than 1%).[8,38] The prognosis of SH-I and SH-II is the best, followed by SH-III and then SH-IV. This prognosis is thought to corre-late with the magnitude of initial traumatic force and the resultant physeal injury. The strength of the physis is reduced at the metaphyseal junction compared to the epiph-yseal junction, making SH-II the most common physeal fracture type. SH-VI has also been proposed as an open fracture with partial physis loss.[37]

1. SH-I (**Fig. 1**A): It only involves the physis, with slight physeal widening or translation that may not be obvious in plain films.
2. SH-II (**Fig. 1**B, C): The fracture line extends from the physis into the metaphysis.
3. SH-III (**Fig. 2**): The fracture line extends from the physis into the epiphysis.
4. SH-IV (**Fig. 3**): The fracture line extends from the physis into both the metaphysis and the epiphysis.
5. SH-V: It is a crush injury to the physis (rarely seen).

Transitional Fractures

Patients between 12 and 15 years of age with closing physes are susceptible to spe-cific distal tibial fracture patterns. The Tillaux fracture (**Fig. 4**A, B) is a variant of SH-III

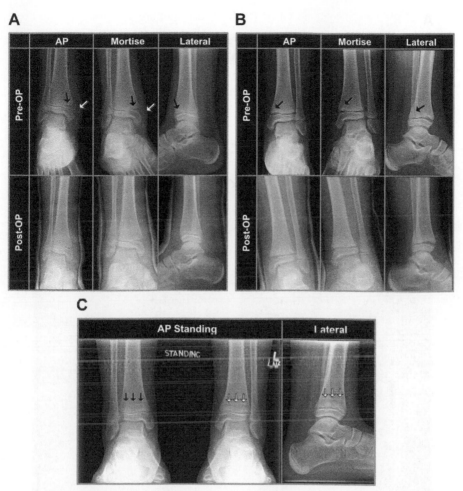

Fig. 1. (*A*) Salter-Harris Type I fracture. Note the widening of the physis at the medial side of distal tibia (*black arrows*) and the adjacent soft tissue swelling (*white arrows*), even though no obvious fracture lines were seen. (*B*) Salter-Harris Type II fracture. The fracture line extended into the metaphysis (*black arrows*) and was seen clearly in the lateral view. Casting resulted in satisfactory outcome in both patients. (*C*) Park-Harris line (*white arrows*) symmetric to the uninjured ankle (*black arrows*) and parallel to the physis with longitudinal growth at one year follow-up, indicating restoration of normal physeal growth. AP, anteroposterior; Post-OP, postoperative; Pre-OP, preoperative.

fractures and represents avulsion of anterolateral distal tibia epiphysis at the insertion site of anterior inferior tibiofibular ligament. This fracture accounts for less than 5% of pediatric ankle fractures and may present together with a distal fibula fracture. Triplane fractures (**Fig. 4**C, D) are complex, 3-dimensional SH-IV fractures, occurring in younger children than the Tillaux fractures. In younger adolescents, more of the distal tibial physis is open and vulnerable to mechanical failure through multiple planes. By definition, there are fracture lines in 3 planes: coronal, sagittal, and axial (transverse). The classic ones are lateral and medial triplane fractures. Lateral triplane fractures are the most common, with fracture lines in the tibia metaphysis (coronal),

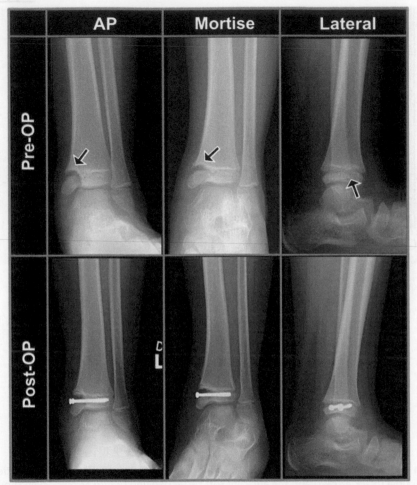

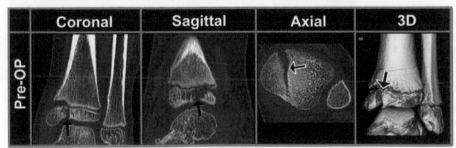

Fig. 2. (*A*) Salter-Harris Type III fracture with a displaced medial tibial epiphyseal fragment (*black arrows*) was treated by open reduction with two parallel cannulated screws fixation. (*B*) CT scan excluded extension of the fracture into the tibial metaphysis and confirmed the Salter-Harris Type III diagnosis. 3D, 3-dimensional; AP, anteroposterior; Post-OP, postoperative; Pre-OP, preoperative.

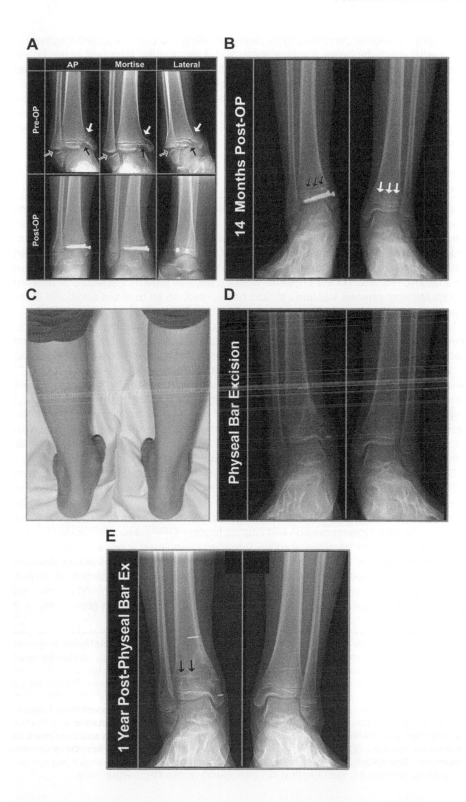

the epiphysis (sagittal), and the physis (axial), resulting in 3 parts: a spiked fragment in the medial epi-metaphysis, the tibia shaft, and a rectangular fragment in the lateral epiphysis. This can present as a 2-part fracture if the tibia shaft is not separated with the epi-metaphysis fragment. Medial triplane fractures are less common, with fracture lines in the tibia epiphysis (coronal), the metaphysis (sagittal), and the physis (axial). Intramalleolar fractures are triplane variants and can be subcategorized into intra-articular and extra-articular types.[39] A CT may be helpful to determine whether the fracture is intra-articular or displaced.

TREATMENT STRATEGIES
General Concepts and Principles of Treatment

The long-term treatment aims are to minimize angular deformity and leg-length discrepancy, to avoid posttraumatic arthritis, and to achieve normal ankle function. Intra-articular fractures should be reduced anatomically to restore joint surface congruency and to correct angular limb deformity. Articular step-off should be less than 1 to 2 mm.[40] In growing children with open physes, efforts should be made to achieve an anatomic reduction of the physis to facilitate physeal growth. Repeated or delayed manipulation of physeal fractures should be avoided, so as to avoid additional damage to the physis with incurrent risks of premature closure.[38,41]

Nondisplaced fractures can be treated with a cast. Weight-bearing status and duration of the immobilization depends on the fracture type and stability. Low-risk ankle fractures, such as distal fibular avulsion fractures, nondisplaced fibular SH-I fractures, or lateral talus avulsion fractures, may be treated in an air splint or walking boot.[42-44] SH-I distal fibular fractures may be far less common than previously thought. A recent report of 18 patients with SH-I fractures who underwent research MRI revealed intact physis in 100% and ligament injury in 90% of all cases.[45] Physeal arrest after nondisplaced fibula fractures has not been reported in the literature, furthering the support for expectant management of these fracture patterns with immediate weight-bearing as tolerated and immobilization as needed for comfort.[46]

Simple displaced tibia and fibula fractures can be managed with closed reduction (CR) and casting. Unstable fracture patterns may require percutaneous fixation or open reduction if a satisfactory CR cannot be maintained. A long leg cast with the knee flexed will add rotational stability and may prevent displacement after successful closed reduction. Open reduction and internal fixation (ORIF) is recommended for displaced intra-articular fractures. Partially threaded cannulated screws or smooth pins are used for internal fixation, although adolescents with extensile fracture patterns may occasionally need a plate-screw construct. Percutaneous insertion of screws and pins is used when possible. Implants that cross the physis should be avoided when possible in skeletally immature patients, as they may result in growth arrest. If

Fig. 3. (A) Salter-Harris Type IV fracture with a displaced medial tibial epiphyseal fragment (*black arrows*) and a posteromedial metaphyseal fragment (*white arrows*), treated by open reduction with cannulated screw fixation. Also note the widening and translation at the distal fibular physis (*grey arrows*) implicating a Salter-Harris Type I fracture. (B) Follow up of the Salter-Harris TypeIV fracture in (A) revealed progressive angular deformity, with Park-Harris growth arrest lines (*black arrows*) that is not symmetric to the normal side (*white arrows*). (C) Clinical photo showing varus deformity of the hindfoot on the right. (D) Physeal bar resection and cranioplast interposition were performed with radiolucent bone markers to monitor growth. (E) One year following physeal bar resection, a Park-Harris growth resumption line (*black arrows*) is now visible and the right distal tibial physis has grown. AP, anteroposterior; Ex, excision; Post-OP, postoperative; Pre-OP, preoperative.

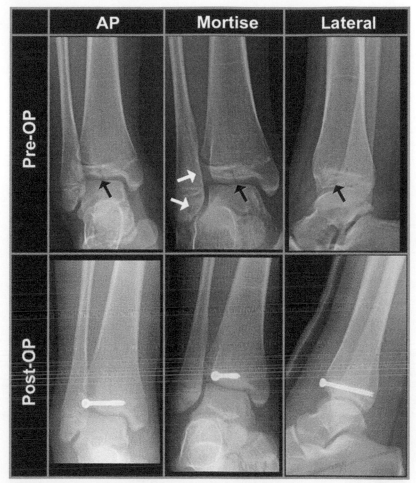

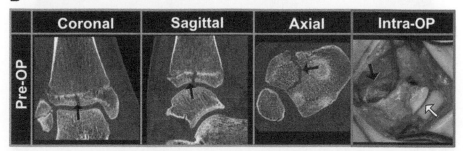

Fig. 4. (*A*) Juvenile Tillaux fracture with an avulsion of lateral tibial epiphysis (*black arrows*) was treated by open reduction with cannulated screw fixation. Also note the co-existing Salter-Harris Type IV distal fibular fracture (*white arrows*) (*B*) CT scan confirmed the diagnosis of Tillaux fracture (*black arrows*) and showed that the physis is closed in the medial side of distal tibia. The tibio-talar joint was visualized during surgery (*white arrows*) (*C*) Triplane fracture with coronal fracture line (*black arrows*) in both epiphysis and metaphysis, axial fracture line in the physis as well as metaphyseal fracture line in the sagittal plane (*white arrows*) around the distal tibial epiphysis (*dashed circle*), as clearly identified in (*D*) CT scan. AP, anteroposterior; Intra-OP, intraoperative; Post-OP, postoperative; Pre-OP, preoperative.

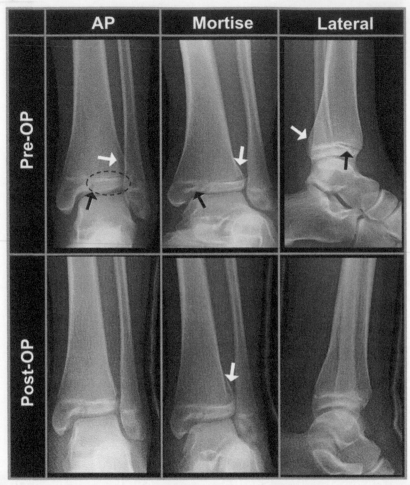

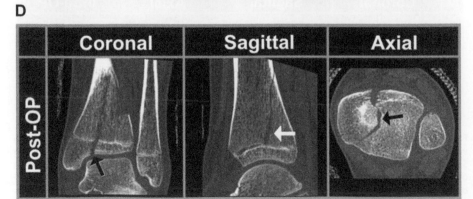

Fig. 4. (*continued*)

fixation across the physis is inevitable in children with open physes, use only smooth pins instead of screws or threaded wires and plan for early removal postoperatively.

Screw removal may be offered for symptomatic implants, but delayed removal of partially threaded screws may be difficult. Some investigators favor the use of bio-absorbable screws for epiphyseal fixation, which obviates removal and may have less effect on joint contact forces and articular pressures compared with metal implants.[47,48] In the authors' clinical practice, however, they favor metal implants for ease of use and perceived improved purchase. Screws are removed electively as indicated by patient symptoms.

Management of Displaced Physeal Fractures

Significant physeal fractures are typically managed with 6 weeks of non-weight-bearing. Anatomic alignment should be restored with closed or open reduction as needed if there is interposed periosteum or a block to reduction. CR may be successful for SH-I and SH-II fracture patterns. Displaced SH-III and SH-IV fracture patterns benefit from anatomic reduction, internal fixation, and restoration of joint space congruity. Surgical fixation has been associated with a lower rate of physeal arrest following these fractures compared with CR alone.[49] In the case of open reduction, it is important to avoid extensive dissection or periosteal stripping at the physis, as this may contribute to premature physeal arrest.

Displaced Tillaux and triplane fractures may be treated with attempted CR. CR for a Tillaux fracture entails plantar flexion and internal rotation and manual pressure over the displaced fragment. Triplane fractures may be reduced with axial traction and internal rotation. A long leg cast is applied with the foot internally rotated. A CT is best obtained after CR to assess the adequacy of alignment and whether surgical management is necessary. If the reduction is satisfactory, weekly radiographs should be obtained to ensure maintenance of alignment for 3 weeks, at which point the child can be transitioned to a short-leg, non-weight-bearing cast for an additional 3 weeks. If the articular alignment is not anatomic, ORIF is recommended.

Displaced distal fibula fractures frequently accompany distal tibial fractures but can also present in isolation. In contrast to isolated distal tibial fractures, there is a very low risk of isolated fibular growth physeal arrest.[46] For displaced fibular fracture associated with a tibia fracture, reduction of the tibial fracture usually results in reduction of the fibula as well. Occasionally a greenstick or displaced fibula fracture will block reduction of the distal tibia fracture, in which case closed or open reduction of the fibula may be necessary. In cases with the need for additional stability, pinning of the fibula usually provides sufficient fixation.

COMPLICATIONS

Maintenance of bony alignment, joint space congruency, and restoration of physeal anatomy are the primary concerns in the early follow-up period. During the midterm to long-term follow-up periods, patients with growth remaining may require monitoring for growth arrest and subsequent angular deformity or leg-length discrepancy.

For patients at high risk of growth arrest, a baseline scanogram and hand bone age may be helpful to confirm an arrest and to predict anticipated growth remaining and projected leg-length discrepancy at skeletal maturity.

Growth Disturbance

The overall risk of premature physeal closure ranges from 2% to 67% for SH-I and SH-II fractures and 8% to 50% for SH-III and SH-IV fractures.[12,38,41,49,50] Fracture type, high-energy trauma, higher initial displacement, and multiple manipulation attempts are associated with growth arrest.[38] Barmada and colleagues[41] found higher rates of physeal arrest (60% vs 17%) if a residual gap greater than 3 mm was seen at the physis for SH-I and II fracture patterns and recommended open reduction to remove entrapped periosteum in these settings.

High-risk patients are followed for several years until normative growth of the physis is established. Symmetric Park-Harris growth resumption lines will show restoration of physeal growth (see **Fig. 1**C). In contrast, Park-Harris growth arrest lines that are incomplete or tracked to the physis indicates physeal bar formation (see **Fig. 3**B). Complete growth arrest can result in leg-length discrepancy without angular deformity, whereas partial growth arrest may cause progressive angular deformity.[51] The treatment of complete growth arrest depends on the expected remaining growth of the distal tibia and the extent of physeal bar, typically measured on CT. If the remaining growth is less than 1 cm, nonoperative management may be fine. If the remaining growth is more than 1 cm or the child has more than 3 years of growth remaining, physeal bar excision can be performed if less than 50% of the physis is involved. If there is less than 3 years of growth remaining and there is a progressive leg-length discrepancy and/or angular deformity, tibial and fibular epiphyseodesis may be performed to prevent progression of the deformity. Contralateral epiphyseodesis may also be considered to prevent worsening leg-length discrepancy until the completion of skeletal growth. If more than 50% of the physis is involved and the predicted leg-length discrepancy is significant, future limb-lengthening surgery may be discussed. Attempted physeal bar resection may be indicated in the very young child, as it is significantly less morbid than a limb-lengthening procedure.

Angular deformity from physeal arrest or malunion may alter the ankle joint biomechanics and ankle range of motion and increase joint contact stress, resulting in early arthritis. Angular deformity from malunion remote from the physis can be treated with guided growth/temporary epiphyseodesis plates if patients are skeletally immature with sufficient growth remaining. Guided growth should not be attempted in conjunction with physeal bar resection at the same physis because of the risks of excessive tethering of the growth plate. For severe angular deformity, corrective procedures, such as osteotomy, may be performed either in isolation or at the time of physeal bar resection. The acceptable range of angular deformity and indication for surgical correction has not been well established. Children with isolated or combined angulation of 5° in the coronal or 10° in the sagittal plane[12,52] may remain clinically asymptomatic and fully functional in daily activities but may be at an increased risk of arthritis in adulthood.

Ankle Joint Problems

Intra-articular ankle fractures may predispose patients to future ankle arthritis, stiffness, and persistent pain. SH-III and SH-IV distal tibial fractures carry higher risks of posttraumatic arthritis. In a series of 68 patients with an average 27 years of follow-up, 11.8% of patients developed radiographic signs of ankle arthritis, most commonly associated with persistent varus or valgus angular deformity of 5° or more.[51] Overall, 29% of all patients with SH-III and SH-IV developed radiographic signs of ankle arthritis.[51] The risk of ankle arthritis is decreased by anatomic reduction.[53] Stiffness may be addressed with physical therapy and rehabilitation programs. MRI can be considered for persistent mechanical symptoms, which may indicate osteochondral lesions. Reflex sympathetic dystrophy, also known as complex regional pain syndrome, is a rare but frustrating complication after ankle injury; the prevalence is higher in young girls than boys.[54] The treatment is limited to physical and psychological therapies, although most pediatric patients note symptom improvement over time.

SUMMARY AND FUTURE DIRECTIONS

The general concepts and principles of the treatment of pediatric ankle fractures are similar to those for other pediatric physeal injuries. Treatment of premature physeal closure focuses on addressing the resultant angular deformity or LLD. Future direction may involve a biological solution to salvage or resume the viability of the injured growth plate. Successful outcomes depend on early recognition and treatment of specific pediatric ankle fracture patterns.

REFERENCES

1. Rohmiller MT, Gaynor TP, Pawelek J, et al. Salter-Harris I and II fractures of the distal tibia: does mechanism of injury relate to premature physeal closure? J Pediatr Orthop 2006;26:322–8.
2. Landin LA, Danielsson LG. Children's ankle fractures. Classification and epidemiology. Acta Orthop Scand 1983;54:634–40.
3. Peterson HA, Madhok R, Benson JT, et al. Physeal fractures: part 1. Epidemiology in Olmsted County, Minnesota, 1979–1988. J Pediatr Orthop 1994;14: 423–30.
4. Peterson CA, Peterson HA. Analysis of the incidence of injuries to the epiphyseal growth plate. J Trauma 1972;12:275–81.
5. Mizuta T, Benson WM, Foster BK, et al. Statistical analysis of the incidence of physeal injuries. J Pediatr Orthop 1987;7:518–23.
6. McHugh MP. Oversized young athletes: a weighty concern. Br J Sports Med 2010;44:45–9.
7. Zonfrillo MR, Seiden JA, House EM, et al. The association of overweight and ankle injuries in children. Ambul Pediatr 2008;8:66–9.
8. Spiegel PG, Cooperman DR, Laros GS. Epiphyseal fractures of the distal ends of the tibia and fibula. A retrospective study of two hundred and thirty-seven cases in children. J Bone Joint Surg Am 1978;60:1046–50.
9. Goldberg VM, Aadalen R. Distal tibial epiphyseal injuries: the role of athletics in 53 cases. Am J Sports Med 1978;6:263–8.
10. Aslam N, Gwilym S, Apostolou C, et al. Microscooter injuries in the paediatric population. Eur J Emerg Med 2004;11:148–50.
11. Fong DT, Man CY, Yung PS, et al. Sport-related ankle injuries attending an accident and emergency department. Injury 2008;39:1222–7.
12. Langenskiold A. Traumatic premature closure of the distal tibial epiphyseal plate. Acta Orthop Scand 1967;38:520–31.
13. Salter RB. Injuries of the ankle in children. Orthop Clin North Am 1974;5: 147–52.
14. Hajdu S, Schwendenwein E, Kaltenecker G, et al. Growth potential of different zones of the growth plate-an experimental study in rabbits. J Orthop Res 2012; 30:162–8.
15. Hajdu S, Schwendenwein E, Kaltenecker G, et al. The effect of drilling and screw fixation of the growth plate-an experimental study in rabbits. J Orthop Res 2011; 29:1834–9.
16. Beals RK, Skyhar M. Growth and development of the tibia, fibula, and ankle joint. Clin Orthop Relat Res 1984;(182):289–92.

17. Hansman CF. Appearance and fusion of ossification centers in the human skeleton. Am J Roentgenol Radium Ther Nucl Med 1962;88:476–82.
18. Ogden JA, McCarthy SM. Radiology of postnatal skeletal development. VIII. Distal tibia and fibula. Skeletal Radiol 1983;10:209–20.
19. Ogden JA, Lee J. Accessory ossification patterns and injuries of the malleoli. J Pediatr Orthop 1990;10:306–16.
20. Mellado JM, Ramos A, Salvado E, et al. Accessory ossicles and sesamoid bones of the ankle and foot: imaging findings, clinical significance and differential diagnosis. Eur Radiol 2003;13(Suppl 6):L164–77.
21. Pritchett JW. Growth and growth prediction of the fibula. Clin Orthop Relat Res 1997;(334):251–6.
22. King J, Diefendorf D, Apthorp J, et al. Analysis of 429 fractures in 189 battered children. J Pediatr Orthop 1988;8:585–9.
23. Stiell I, Wells G, Laupacis A, et al. Multicentre trial to introduce the Ottawa ankle rules for use of radiography in acute ankle injuries. Multicentre Ankle Rule Study Group. BMJ 1995;311:594–7.
24. Dowling S, Spooner CH, Liang Y, et al. Accuracy of Ottawa ankle rules to exclude fractures of the ankle and midfoot in children: a meta-analysis. Acad Emerg Med 2009;16:277–87.
25. Dowling SK, Wishart I. Use of the Ottawa ankle rules in children: a survey of physicians' practice patterns. CJEM 2011;13:333–8. E344–6.
26. Lucchesi GM, Jackson RE, Peacock WF, et al. Sensitivity of the Ottawa rules. Ann Emerg Med 1995;26:1–5.
27. Crosswell S, Leaman A, Phung W. Minimising negative ankle and foot X-rays in the emergency department-are the Ottawa ankle rules good enough? Injury 2014;45:2002–4.
28. Boutis K, von Keyserlingk C, Willan A, et al. Cost consequence analysis of implementing the low risk ankle rule in emergency departments. Ann Emerg Med 2015. [Epub ahead of print].
29. Boutis K, Komar L, Jaramillo D, et al. Sensitivity of a clinical examination to predict need for radiography in children with ankle injuries: a prospective study. Lancet 2001;358:2118–21.
30. Liporace FA, Yoon RS, Kubiak EN, et al. Does adding computed tomography change the diagnosis and treatment of Tillaux and triplane pediatric ankle fractures? Orthopedics 2012;35:e208–12.
31. Petit P, Panuel M, Faure F, et al. Acute fracture of the distal tibial physis: role of gradient-echo MR imaging versus plain film examination. AJR Am J Roentgenol 1996;166:1203–6.
32. Lohman M, Kivisaari A, Kallio P, et al. Acute paediatric ankle trauma: MRI versus plain radiography. Skeletal Radiol 2001;30:504–11.
33. Gill JB, Risko T, Raducan V, et al. Comparison of manual and gravity stress radiographs for the evaluation of supination-external rotation fibular fractures. J Bone Joint Surg Am 2007;89:994–9.
34. Schock HJ, Pinzur M, Manion L, et al. The use of gravity or manual-stress radiographs in the assessment of supination-external rotation fractures of the ankle. J Bone Joint Surg Br 2007;89:1055–9.
35. Salter RB. Injuries of the epiphyseal plate. Instr Course Lect 1992;41:351–9.
36. Peterson HA. Physeal fractures: part 3. Classification. J Pediatr Orthop 1994;14:439–48.
37. Peterson HA. Physeal fractures: part 2. Two previously unclassified types. J Pediatr Orthop 1994;14:431–8.

38. Leary JT, Handling M, Talerico M, et al. Physeal fractures of the distal tibia: predictive factors of premature physeal closure and growth arrest. J Pediatr Orthop 2009;29:356–61.
39. Shin AY, Moran ME, Wenger DR. Intramalleolar triplane fractures of the distal tibial epiphysis. J Pediatr Orthop 1997;17:352–5.
40. Crawford AH. Triplane and Tillaux fractures: is a 2 mm residual gap acceptable? J Pediatr Orthop 2012;32(Suppl 1):S69–73.
41. Barmada A, Gaynor T, Mubarak SJ. Premature physeal closure following distal tibia physeal fractures: a new radiographic predictor. J Pediatr Orthop 2003; 23:733–9.
42. Barnett PL, Lee MH, Oh L, et al. Functional outcome after air-stirrup ankle brace or fiberglass backslab for pediatric low-risk ankle fractures: a randomized observer-blinded controlled trial. Pediatr Emerg Care 2012;28:745–9.
43. Boutis K, Willan AR, Babyn P, et al. A randomized, controlled trial of a removable brace versus casting in children with low-risk ankle fractures. Pediatrics 2007; 119:e1256–63.
44. Gleeson AP, Stuart MJ, Wilson B, et al. Ultrasound assessment and conservative management of inversion injuries of the ankle in children: plaster of Paris versus Tubigrip. J Bone Joint Surg Br 1996;78:484–7.
45. Boutis K, Narayanan UG, Dong FF, et al. Magnetic resonance imaging of clinically suspected Salter-Harris I fracture of the distal fibula. Injury 2010;41:852–6.
46. Peterson HA. Epiphyseal growth plate fractures. Leipzig (Germany): Springer; 2007.
47. Podeszwa DA, Wilson PL, Holland AR, et al. Comparison of bioabsorbable versus metallic implant fixation for physeal and epiphyseal fractures of the distal tibia. J Pediatr Orthop 2008;28:859–63.
48. Charlton M, Costello R, Mooney JF 3rd, et al. Ankle joint biomechanics following transepiphyseal screw fixation of the distal tibia. J Pediatr Orthop 2005;25: 635–40.
49. Cass JR, Peterson HA. Salter-Harris type-IV injuries of the distal tibial epiphyseal growth plate, with emphasis on those involving the medial malleolus. J Bone Joint Surg Am 1983;65:1059–70.
50. Kling TF Jr, Bright RW, Hensinger RN. Distal tibial physeal fractures in children that may require open reduction. J Bone Joint Surg Am 1984;66:647–57.
51. Caterini R, Farsetti P, Ippolito E. Long-term follow-up of physeal injury to the ankle. Foot Ankle 1991;11:372–83.
52. McDonnell TC, Sullivan TJ, Hessburg PF, et al. Steady-state sulfur critical loads and exceedances for protection of aquatic ecosystems in the U.S. Southern Appalachian Mountains. J Environ Manage 2014;146:407–19.
53. Ertl JP, Barrack RL, Alexander AH, et al. Triplane fracture of the distal tibial epiphysis. Long-term follow-up. J Bone Joint Surg Am 1988;70:967–76.
54. Wilder RT, Berde CB, Wolohan M, et al. Reflex sympathetic dystrophy in children. Clinical characteristics and follow-up of seventy patients. J Bone Joint Surg Am 1992;74:910–9.

Index

Note: Page numbers of article titles are in **boldface** type.

http://dx.doi.org/10.1016/S1083-7515(15)00110-2
1083-7515/15/$ – see front matter © 2015 Elsevier Inc. All rights reserved.

United States
Postal Service

Statement of Ownership, Management, and Circulation
(All Periodicals Publications Except Requestor Publications)

1. Publication Title	2. Publication Number	3. Filing Date
Foot and Ankle Clinics of North America	0 1 6 - 3 6 8	9/18/15

4. Issue Frequency	5. Number of Issues Published Annually	6. Annual Subscription Price
Mar, Jun, Sep, Dec	4	$330.00

7. Complete Mailing Address of Known Office of Publication (Not printer) (Street, city, county, state, and ZIP+4®)

Elsevier Inc.
360 Park Avenue South
New York, NY 10010-1710

Contact Person
Stephen R. Bushing

Telephone (Include area code)
215-239-3688

8. Complete Mailing Address of Headquarters or General Business Office of Publisher (Not printer)

Elsevier Inc., 360 Park Avenue South, New York, NY 10010-1710

9. Full Names and Complete Mailing Addresses of Publisher, Editor, and Managing Editor (Do not leave blank)

Publisher (Name and complete mailing address)

Linda Belfus, Elsevier Inc., 1600 John F. Kennedy Blvd., Suite 1800, Philadelphia, PA 19103

Editor (Name and complete mailing address)

Jennifer Flynn-Briggs, Elsevier Inc., 1600 John F. Kennedy Blvd., Suite 1800, Philadelphia, PA 19103-2899

Managing Editor (Name and complete mailing address)

Adrianne Brigido, Elsevier Inc., 1600 John F. Kennedy Blvd., Suite 1800, Philadelphia, PA 19103-2899

10. Owner (Do not leave blank. If the publication is owned by a corporation, give the name and address of the corporation immediately followed by the names and addresses of all stockholders owning or holding 1 percent or more of the total amount of stock. If not owned by a corporation, give the names and addresses of the individual owners. If owned by a partnership or other unincorporated firm, give its name and address as well as those of each individual owner. If the publication is published by a nonprofit organization, give its name and address.)

Full Name	Complete Mailing Address
Wholly owned subsidiary of	1600 John F. Kennedy Blvd. Ste. 1800
Reed/Elsevier, US holdings	Philadelphia, PA 19103-2899

11. Known Bondholders, Mortgagees, and Other Security Holders Owning or Holding 1 Percent or More of Total Amount of Bonds, Mortgages, or Other Securities. If none, check box ☐ None

Full Name	Complete Mailing Address
N/A	

12. Tax Status (For completion by nonprofit organizations authorized to mail at nonprofit rates) (Check one)
The purpose, function, and nonprofit status of this organization and the exempt status for federal income tax purposes:
☐ Has Not Changed During Preceding 12 Months
☐ Has Changed During Preceding 12 Months (Publisher must submit explanation of change with this statement)

13. Publication Title	14. Issue Date for Circulation Data Below
Foot and Ankle Clinics of North America	September 2015

15. Extent and Nature of Circulation			Average No. Copies Each Issue During Preceding 12 Months	No. Copies of Single Issue Published Nearest to Filing Date
a. Total Number of Copies (Net press run)			721	568
b. Legitimate Paid and/or Requested Distribution (By Mail and Outside the Mail)	(1)	Mailed Outside County Paid/Requested Mail Subscriptions stated on PS Form 3541. (Include paid distribution above nominal rate, advertiser's proof copies and exchange copies)	409	322
	(2)	Mailed In-County Paid/Requested Mail Subscriptions stated on PS Form 3541. (Include paid distribution above nominal rate, advertiser's proof copies and exchange copies)		
	(3)	Paid Distribution Outside the Mails Including Sales Through Dealers And Carriers, Street Vendors, Counter Sales, and Other Paid Distribution Outside USPS®	121	123
	(4)	Paid Distribution by Other Classes of Mail Through the USPS (e.g. First-Class Mail®)		
c. Total Paid and or Requested Circulation (Sum of 15b (1), (2), (3), and (4))			530	445
d. Free or Nominal Rate Distribution (By Mail and Outside the Mail)	(1)	Free or Nominal Rate Outside-County Copies included on PS Form 3541	28	20
	(2)	Free or Nominal Rate In-County Copies included on PS Form 3541		
	(3)	Free or Nominal Rate Copies mailed at Other classes Through the USPS (e.g. First-Class Mail®)		
	(4)	Free or Nominal Rate Distribution Outside the Mail (Carriers or Other means)		
e. Total Nonrequested Distribution (Sum of 15d (1), (2), (3) and (4))			28	20
f. Total Distribution (Sum of 15c and 15e)			558	465
g. Copies not Distributed (See instructions to publishers #4 (page #3))			163	103
h. Total (Sum of 15f and g)			721	568
i. Percent Paid and/or Requested Circulation (15c divided by 15f times 100)			94.98%	95.70%

16. Electronic Copy Circulation	Average No. Copies Each Issue During Preceding 12 Months	No. Copies of Single Issue Published Nearest to Filing Date
a. Paid Electronic Copies		
b. Total paid Print Copies (Line 15c) + Paid Electronic copies (Line 16a)		
c. Total Print Distribution (Line 15f) + Paid Electronic Copies (Line 16a)		
d. Percent Paid (Both Print & Electronic copies) (16b divided by 16c X 100)		

☐ If present, claiming electronic copies go to line 16 on page 3. If you are not claiming Electronic copies, skip to line 17 on page 3.

☐ I certify that 50% of all my distributed copies (electronic and print) are paid above a nominal price.

17. Publication of Statement of Ownership
☐ If the publication is a general publication, publication of this statement is required. Will be printed in the December 2015 issue of this publication.

18. Signature and Title of Editor, Publisher, Business Manager, or Owner

Stephen R. Bushing

Stephen R. Bushing – Inventory Distribution Coordinator

Date
September 18, 2015

I certify that all information furnished on this form is true and complete. I understand that anyone who furnishes false or misleading information on this form or who omits material or information requested on the form may be subject to criminal sanctions (including fines and imprisonment) and/or civil sanctions (including civil penalties).

PS Form 3526, July 2014 (Page 3 of 3) (Instructions Page 3) PSN 7530-01-000-9931 PRIVACY NOTICE: See our Privacy policy in www.usps.com

PS Form 3526, July 2014 (Page 1 of 3 (Instructions Page 3))

Printed and bound by CPI Group (UK) Ltd, Croydon, CR0 4YY

03/10/2024

01040488-0017